WITHDRAWN by
Memphis Public Library

NewHope
FOR PEOPLE WITH

Weight Problems

Other Books in Prima's NEW HOPE Series

New Hope for People with Alzheimer's and Their Caregivers

New Hope for People with Bipolar Disorder

New Hope for People with Depression

New Hope for People with Diabetes

New Hope for People with Fibromyalgia

New Hope for People with Lupus

New Hope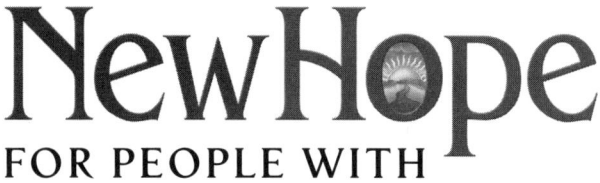
FOR PEOPLE WITH
Weight Problems

Lawrence J. Cheskin, M.D.,
and Ron Sauder

Foreword by Benjamin Caballero, M.D., Ph.D.

PRIMA PUBLISHING

Copyright © 2002 by Prima Publishing, a division of Random House, Inc.

All rights reserved. No part of this book may be reproduced or transmitted in any form or by any means, electronic or mechanical, including photocopying, recording, or by any information storage or retrieval system, without written permission from Random House, Inc., except for the inclusion of brief quotations in a review.

Published by Prima Publishing, Roseville, California. Member of the Crown Publishing Group, a division of Random House, Inc.

PRIMA PUBLISHING and colophon are trademarks of Random House, Inc., registered with the United States Patent and Trademark Office.

In order to protect their privacy, the names of some individuals cited in this book have been changed.

Warning—Disclaimer

This book is not intended to provide medical advice and is sold with the understanding that the publisher and the author are not liable for the misconception or misuse of information provided. The author and Random House shall have neither liability nor responsibility to any person or entity with respect to any loss, damage, or injury caused or alleged to be caused directly or indirectly by the information contained in this book or the use of any products mentioned. Readers should not use any of the products discussed in this book without the advice of a medical professional.

Interior design by Peri Poloni, Knockout Design
Illustrations by Laurie Baker-McNeile

Library of Congress Cataloging-in-Publication Data

Cheskin, Lawrence J.
  New hope for people with weight problems : your friendly, authoritative guide to the latest in traditional and complementary solutions / Lawrence J. Cheskin, Ron Sauder.
    p. cm.—(New hope series)
  Includes biographical references and index.
  ISBN 0-7615-1160-1
  1. Weight loss—Popular works. I. Sauder, Ron. II. Title.
RM222.2 .C475 2002
613.7—dc21   2002016974

02 03 04 05 HH 10 9 8 7 6 5 4 3 2 1
Printed in the United States of America

First Edition

Visit us online at www.primapublishing.com

To my parents, Greta and Al Cheskin

—L.C.

To Debbie, Katie, and Andrew

—R.S.

Contents

Foreword by Benjamin Caballero, M.D., Ph.D. ix
Acknowledgments xi

1. What Is Obesity? 1

2. Diagnosis: Getting Some Answers 35

3. Diet and Exercise: Can You Lose Weight Without Them? 69

4. Drug Treatment for Weight Loss 109

5. Surgery: Last Chance or Best Prospect? 129

6. Complementary and Alternative Treatments 161

7. Family, Society, and Our Overweight Kids 187

8. On the Horizon 219

Appendix: Resources 243
Notes 247
Glossary 263
Index 267

Foreword

THERE IS ONE indisputable fact about obesity: Excess body weight is one of the most serious public health problems in the United States. As described in these pages, almost two of every three adult Americans weigh more than they should, and thus have an increased risk for several conditions, including diabetes, hypertension, and cardiovascular disease.

It is thus not surprising that there are as many books about weight control as there are "diet" foods in the supermarket. Millions of people are trying to lose weight, even many who don't need to. And all are searching for the "magic potion": a plan that will allow you to lose weight and eat as much as you like, gain muscle and lose fat while watching TV, and so on. Regretfully, after a few weeks, you will realize that the only thing you really lost was the money you paid for the book.

Larry Cheskin and Ron Sauder have a different approach. They are not out to sell you a program; their intention is to empower you to choose what is best for you and to do so with as clear an understanding of your options as possible. First, they provide in simple but accurate language, up-to-date information on recent scientific findings on the causes of overweight and obesity (in fact, the first section of the book is a very useful guide to navigating the daily flood of information we receive from the media on diet, weight, and health). Next, they review current weight-loss approaches, including diet programs, pharmacological treatments, surgery, and alternative treatments such as acupuncture and herbal medicine. These methods are discussed in an objective, clear language, with the authors always providing a "take home message" regarding their potential effectiveness for each individual situation. The authors clearly succeed in their efforts to make complex scientific concepts understandable for the general public. The inclusion of case studies is particularly useful to understand what we can do to maintain healthy body weight at different life stages.

You will find no magic potion in this book. Instead, you will get clear and objective information on current scientific trends on weight management and a detailed description of weight-control options that may best suit your particular situation. This book is essential not only for those contemplating a weight-loss plan, but also for health professionals involved in weight management. And, by helping people make considered, informed choices regarding their body weight, this book certainly gives us all *new hope*.

                Benjamin Caballero, M.D., Ph.D.
                Director, Center for Human Nutrition
                Johns Hopkins University

Acknowledgments

WE WOULD LIKE to thank the many people who freely shared their time and expertise with us in the course of preparing this book.

In 12 years as director of the Johns Hopkins Weight Management Center, one of us [Dr. Cheskin] has been privileged to witness firsthand the struggles of many hundreds of individuals as they battled against the often painful burden of obesity. It is on the basis of this experience—and of the patients' myriad individual stories—that we can state emphatically that obese people are not lazy, self-indulgent, or mentally ill, at least not to any greater degree than we are as a whole. To the contrary, most are motivated, realistic, and hardworking. But obesity is an excruciating medical condition to overcome, as this book makes clear.

Both of us, as coauthors, would like to express our appreciation to those persons identified as Linda Cartwright, Joanna Givens, and Melissa Humphreys, whose lifelong battles against overweight are profiled in this book. They are brave, articulate, and good-humored. We hope their stories will be inspiring to many who are still summoning up resolve to take the first step on the road to better health. Wayne Smith, a remarkably cheerful evangelist for laparoscopic band weight-loss surgery, also shared generously of his time; his story is summarized in these pages and related in greater detail at www.waynesmith.net.

We owe a special debt to Cynthia Finley, a registered dietitian at the Johns Hopkins Weight Management Center, who contributed the bulk of chapter 3, "Diet and Exercise." She brings to this book some 20 years of experience in working with the special dietary needs of both severely obese and severely malnourished patients at the Johns Hopkins Bayview Medical Center. Her assistance was timely and most welcome. Charles Twilley, a clinical pharmacologist at the Johns Hopkins Bayview Medical Center, contributed dosage and pricing information on the leading anti-obesity drugs.

We would also like to thank the patients and staff at the Johns Hopkins Weight Management Center for their dedication and support.

A number of professionals were helpful in answering questions outside our immediate areas of expertise. We would like to acknowledge the insights and assistance of Dr. Edward Mason, professor emeritus of surgery at the University of Iowa and a giant in the field of obesity surgery; Dr. Thomas Magnuson, director of general surgery at the Johns Hopkins Bayview Medical Center in Baltimore; Dr. Charles Callery, an obesity surgeon in private practice near San Diego, California; Dr. Robert Jackson of Marion, Indiana, the president-elect of the American Academy of Cosmetic Surgery; Dr. Michael Thun, vice president of epidemiology and surveillance research at the American Cancer Society in Atlanta; Dr. Curtiss Cook, an endocrinologist at Emory University in Atlanta; and Dr. Richard C. Niemtzow, an acupuncturist and colonel in the U.S. Air Force, currently based in San Diego, California. Don Mills, communications manager for BioEnterics Corporation in Carpinteria, California, and Steve Adler, vice president of clinical and regulatory affairs at Transneuronix, Inc., provided useful information on their respective companies' research programs.

Georgeann Mallory, executive director at the American Society for Bariatric Surgery, and Morgan Downey, executive director of the American Obesity Association (AOA), answered questions about the activities of their respective groups. We would also like to acknowledge the assistance of Jacqueline Viteri, public relations coordinator at the AOA.

We would like to thank Dr. Donald Saff for his generosity, friendship, and devotion to the future of the Johns Hopkins Weight Management Center. Dr. Benjamin Caballero, of the Johns Hopkins Bloomberg School of Public Health, generously consented to contribute the foreword to this book on the basis of his unsurpassed knowledge of nutrition as a national and international issue.

The project editor of this book, Marjorie Lery, has been a pleasure to work with, serving as a model of tact and diplomacy while keeping us on track in matters large and small; and acquisitions editor Jamie Miller has resolved potential sticking points in a very helpful way. Finally, we would like to thank our families for their gracious acceptance of our sometimes-rude absences during the many hours of research and composition involved in writing a book such as this.

CHAPTER 1

What Is Obesity?

OBESITY IS ALL around us. It is perhaps the most common medical condition in our society. But as common as obesity may be, it has a somewhat uncommon status in the doctor's understanding of health and disease.

First and foremost, there is a strong consensus in the medical profession that excess body weight is bad for our health—and that its effects get steadily worse the more overweight we are. We will review later in this chapter the formidable list of diseases that we can trace to obesity, including its strong connections to heart disease and type 2 diabetes, as well as a growing understanding of its contribution to cancer.

Second, however, it is interesting to note that experts differ on just what obesity *is*. Opinions vary on whether it is more accurate to view obesity as a disease or as a condition with multiple causes that is associated, in turn, with an array of other diseases. Some authorities, such as George Bray of the Pennington Biomedical Research Center at Louisiana State University, state forthrightly that obesity is a *chronic disease* that has been steadily increasing in the United States since World War II. It's also dubbed "a disease in its own right" by the World Health Organization (which, however, perhaps hedging its bets, also refers to obesity as a "complex condition").[1]

The interpretation of obesity as a disease was foreshadowed as long ago as 1757, when a researcher reporting to the Royal Society in London concluded that "corpulency, when to an extraordinary degree, may be reckoned a disease, as it in some measure obstructs the free exercise of the animal functions; and hath a tendency to shorten life, by paving the way to dangerous distempers."[2] Other authorities, such as psychologist Thomas A. Wadden and physician Theodore B. VanItallie, term obesity a *heterogeneous disorder*, with many contributing influences, including people's genes, their bodies' metabolism, and their lifestyles.[3]

> Opinions vary on whether it is more accurate to view obesity as a disease or as a condition with multiple causes that is associated, in turn, with an array of other diseases.

At the Johns Hopkins Weight Management Center, obesity is regarded as a *physical condition* that often has *medical consequences*; obesity must be assessed and treated in an individualized way because the contributing causes vary so widely among different people. Often, a multidisciplinary team consisting of medical doctors, nutritionists, psychologists, and exercise physiologists is needed to achieve the proper assessment and successful long-term treatment of obesity. Peer-to-peer support among patients is also important in achieving weight-loss goals.

Perhaps it is not terribly important to decide, for now, whether obesity is more properly termed a disease, a disorder, or a physical condition. The very fact that these different terms remain in existence should serve to remind us that "overweight" and "obesity" are elusive and slippery concepts. We know them when we see them—especially at the extremes—but they have a whole host of potential causes and a staggering range of potential costs.

A COMPLEX CONDITION

In any discussion of obesity, contradictions abound. Being overweight is, most often, a condition that we create for ourselves. Simply put, we consume more calories than our bodies burn, and the excess has nowhere else to go and is stored as fat (also called *adipose*) tissue.

This simple equation is much more easily described than it is changed. Losing weight permanently is often not just a matter of exercising ordinary amounts of willpower. We will explore the medical, psychological, and cultural factors that may account for this remarkable resistance. Overweight people are often stigmatized as lazy, gluttonous, or self-indulgent. In fact, they are usually none of these things.

Sometimes we are conscious of putting on weight, but more often the pounds simply accumulate over the years without much notice. Rather than originating with some particular germ, gene, or toxin, weight gain in adults is, usually, self-inflicted by our choices and behavior. This does not mean obesity is easy to avoid in our modern culture; in fact, it is so prevalent as to be termed "epidemic" by more than one recent author, both in the United States and, increasingly, worldwide.

Being overweight usually is not the result of a malfunction of a single body system or the impairment of a vital organ. It doesn't result from an infection caused by invading germs, or a tumor caused by cells whose machinery has gone haywire. Nor is it usually a simple product of heredity, although the genes we inherit from our parents can make some of us more likely to gain weight on the abundance of dietary fats and calories we consume in concert with our sedentary culture. Current estimates state that about one-third to one-half of the variations in body fat between individuals may be due to differences in their genetic makeup. But with rare exceptions, obesity does not result from one particular genetic disease or defect. Genes on at least a dozen different chromosomes, by current count, are factors in determining whether laboratory mice grow obese when fed a high-fat diet. It is likely that human obesity will prove to be at least this complex. In any event, genetics

> *Overweight people are often stigmatized as lazy, gluttonous, or self-indulgent. In fact, they are usually none of these things.*

cannot account for the fact that at the time of World War II, only about one in four Americans was overweight or obese, but that today, at least one in two Americans are overweight or obese. To make sense of this veritable gusher of fat over the course of two generations, we must understand what still other writers have termed a "disease of lifestyle"—obesity and overweight as consequences of our modern conveniences, diet, and inactivity. Considered as a public health issue, overweight is overwhelmingly the result of poor eating habits, failure to exercise or work vigorously enough to burn off excess calories, and being surrounded by a culture that supports these bad choices and even *rewards* us for them, usually beginning early in childhood. The following are some of the factors that contribute to obesity and overweight in twentyfirst-century America:

> Considered as a public health issue, overweight is overwhelmingly the result of poor eating habits, failure to exercise or work vigorously enough to burn off excess calories, and being surrounded by a culture that supports these bad choices and even *rewards us for them, usually beginning early in childhood.*

- Too much television—the "couch potato" syndrome
- Not enough vigorous play, exercise, or physical labor
- Too much riding in cars
- Not enough walking or bicycling
- Too much fast food, sodas, snacks, and candy
- Not enough fruits and vegetables
- Too much emotional gratification—or stress relief—from "comfort food" or drink
- Not enough self-control to push away from giant-size restaurant meals and overloaded buffets at every turn

And there are many, many more, which we will review in the course of this book.

These are not easy factors for any of us to change, any more than a fish might find it easy to change the water in which it swims. Changing our *response* to these cultural conditions is at the heart of any successful weight-loss strategy.

If you're overweight, you almost certainly know it—by how hard it is to fasten your slacks over your bulging waistline; by the increasing difficulty you feel in bending over to tie your shoes or climbing out of the bathtub; by the secret way you suck in your stomach when you look sideways in a mirror, trying to catch a glimpse of that svelte reflection you remember from years ago.

If you're obese—a more extreme form of overweight—you know that, too. Odds are you fatigue more easily and have less energy than you did when you weighed less. You likely get out of breath more easily when you are climbing steps or walking to your car. Odds are you have high blood pressure, meaning that your arteries and internal organs are—literally—taking more of a pounding with every heartbeat, putting you at increased risk for kidney damage, heart attack, and stroke. Moreover, odds are your body is beginning to show signs of insulin resistance, a condition that can lead to type 2 diabetes.

> *Changing our response to these cultural conditions is at the heart of any successful weight-loss strategy.*

If you recognize yourself in any of the above—or if you fear that a physical exam would find that you belong to the overweight or even to the obese category—do not despair! First of all, if misery loves company, take comfort in this: *Slightly more than half* of American adults are in the same boat as you. Just look around in the grocery store, the shopping mall, or your office. Statistics may lie, but your eyes won't.

Second, and more important—there's new hope, on a variety of fronts:

- Researchers are gaining new insights into the basis of human motivation and, hence, into how overweight people can avoid relapse and the up-and-down roller-coaster of weight cycling.

- Medical consensus is growing over the essential elements of any diet that will prove healthy and effective in fighting overweight.

- There are new surgical options to the risky—but sometimes necessary—open-gastric bypass operation for the morbidly obese (those who face dramatically higher risks of early death).

- New drugs are being developed as important adjuncts to the fundamental disciplines of exercise and diet.

- Scientists are gaining better insight into the molecular pathways in our brain and body that regulate the intricate balance between appetite, food intake, and a sense of fullness.

- Chemists and food scientists continue to develop fat substitutes such as olestra that are tasty and less damaging to the waistline.

Even Our Pets Are Too Chubby

From portly bulldogs to whip-thin greyhounds, dogs that physically resemble their owners have long been a mainstay of cartoon humor.

These days, it seems, Fido is almost as likely to be rolling side-to-side as he is to be trotting smartly ahead. But, unfortunately, it's not a joke. Anywhere from one-quarter to nearly one-half of our cats and dogs in the United States are obese. The underlying problem is the same as in their human owners—not exercising enough and eating too much.

The dog breeds most prone to obesity are dachshunds, Labrador retrievers, cocker spaniels, beagles, basset hounds, and some Rottweilers, according to Dr. William J. Burkholder, a Texas A&M veterinarian.[4] Like humans, overweight cats and dogs are at risk of heart disease, arthritis, and diabetes, as well as liver problems and bladder cancer.[5]

Neutering or spaying cats and dogs can also make them more prone to obesity, because decreased sex-hormone levels tend to re-

- The Internet has opened a brave new world of "cyber dieting" that has proved to be a promising new strategy for some overweight people.
- Research into "alternative therapies" such as acupuncture and hypnotherapy continues (though with uncertain results).
- There is new hope that as obesity is increasingly recognized as an important worldwide public-health problem, governments will invest more in research into prevention, causes, and treatment of obesity, and that along with this, health-insurance policies will cover the cost of treatment.

In later chapters we will review and explore all of these sources of new hope at greater length. But first, it is important to understand both the known causes of overweight and obesity, as well as the list of

---

duce muscularity and activity levels. Of course, the benefits of neutering far outweigh the possible effects on body weight. And, since a pet's diet is usually totally under our control, weight control is easier to achieve.

The Ralston Purina Company offers the following tips to help your pets stay in fighting trim:

- Cut back on scraps and treats from your table—they are apt to be high in fat and calories. (Unfortunately, it's not usually fruits and vegetables that we're dangling in front of Fido.)
- Give your animal less regular, non-calorie-reduced pet food. Consider switching to a low-calorie, high-fiber food.
- Give your pet more exercise—even if it's only an extra walk or playing catch more.
- Take your pet to the vet for a checkup and weight-reduction plan.[6]

medical conditions that are associated with them and the ill effects that they, in turn, cause.

CAUSES OF OVERWEIGHT AND OBESITY

The root causes—the potential, if you will—of overweight and obesity are programmed into human beings. The *susceptibility* is, literally, in our genes—even if there are comparatively few, and rare, genes that directly cause obesity. From a human evolution standpoint, researchers understand the human capacity for easy weight gain as a positive trait, which was selected by nature because it led to superior survival and reproduction. Now we suffer from the excess of a good thing.

> *From a human evolution standpoint, researchers understand the human capacity for easy weight gain as a positive trait, which was selected by nature because it led to superior survival and reproduction. Now we suffer from the excess of a good thing.*

As long as early humans eked out their living by hunting and gathering, there was never enough food to make people fat—at least not very fat for very long, no more than one season of nature's bounty, perhaps. Individuals who developed the capacity to store reserves of food energy in the form of fat had an obvious advantage in the cold and lean months. Stores of fat were particularly useful for women who were in their childbearing and nursing years. For perhaps 99 percent of the estimated 2 million years of the genus *Homo's* existence, this capacity served our ancestors well. And it *still* does, wherever people live the lifestyle that our genes evolved to support. "There are no reported cases of obesity among current peoples following a hunting and gathering way of life," say anthropologists Peter Brown and Vicki Bentley-Condit.[7]

Beginning with the first stirrings of civilization, though, our distant ancestors' trim lines began to soften. Clay figurines depicting obese women—probably deities—have been dated to the Stone Age period, up to 25,000 years ago. Clay or stone depictions of fleshy

"Mother Goddesses" become even more common with the dawn of agriculture, some 10,000 years ago. References to obesity have been found in every known medical tradition dating back to ancient times, says George Bray, "suggesting that, independent of diet, the potential to store nutrients as fat was selected for by evolution at an early period in human development."[8]

This is part of the historical and cultural backdrop that leads many researchers to view obesity as a disease of lifestyle. The genes that express themselves in varying degrees of overweight are considered to be "susceptibility" genes; they may account for up to one-half the difference in excess weight gained by individuals following the same lifestyle and eating the same diet. However, these dozens of genes, interacting in highly complex ways, cannot begin to account for the rapid acceleration of overweight and obesity that we have seen in the United States since World War II, and especially in the last decade of the 20th century. In a very short period of time, our national waistline has mushroomed much more rapidly than any possible population-wide change in our genetic stock.

The same effects can be seen in the catastrophic changes that often occur to indigenous peoples when they are overtaken by Western society. In his very readable history *Fat: Fighting the Obesity Epidemic*, science writer Robert Pool tells the story of the Pima Indians, a Native American tribe that lived and farmed along the Gila River in what is now southern Arizona. For 19th-century pioneers who survived the hazardous trip west through Apache country, the amicable Pima offered hospitality and refuge. Americans who arrived a century and a half ago in their covered wagons found a hardy people who were "thin and sinewy, their legs chiseled by regular running, their arms strong from the bow, the war club, and the plow."[9] Over the decades, this profile ballooned, as threats from warring tribes disappeared and the Pima became more comfortable and settled. Well-intentioned government programs supplied them with such staples as bacon, cheese, milk, and canned meats, supplanting a traditional, much healthier diet that leaned heavily on cactus buds, wheat, and beans. Today, the average Pima man is 5 feet, 7 inches, and 220 pounds, and some range up to 500 pounds. The average Pima woman is 5 feet, 2.5 inches, and 200 pounds. Diabetes is rampant, striking half of all tribal members over 35 and two-thirds of those reaching 50, giving spawn to cases of blindness, limb amputation, and kidney dialysis.

"The Pimas are the second-fattest group of people in the world," writes Pool, "saved from being the fattest only by the inhabitants of Nauru, an eight-square-mile island in the Western Pacific Ocean whose extensive guano-derived phosphate deposits have made the people of that island some of the wealthiest and most leisurely in the world."

Far from being isolated episodes, these two case studies fall into a recognizable pattern. Obesity is found at rates above the national norm in African Americans, being especially pronounced in the rural South; Native Americans throughout the Southwest; Puerto Ricans and other Hispanic Americans; Gypsies, and Pacific Islanders. Obe-

---

Leading Causes of Obesity

- Lifestyle (overeating, sedentary)
- Genetic diseases and medical disorders

    Cushing's syndrome
    Hypothyroidism
    Polycystic ovary syndrome
    Prader-Willi syndrome
    Disorders of the hypothalamus
    More than 30 other rare disorders and syndromes

- Smoking cessation
- Medications that increase appetite

sity in these ethnic groups can be traced to tangled threads of culture, acculturation to a Western lifestyle, social class, and genetic heritage, according to anthropologists.

When considering the complicated issues of human genetics and obesity, it is wise to bear the following facts in mind:

- We are only in the very early stages of identifying the genes involved in human obesity, much less understanding the ways in which they interact with each other.
- We have no real ability to delete or repair these genes in ways we might desire, even if we could identify them.
- People who may have the same genetic susceptibility can develop very different physiques, depending on how physically active they are, what diet they follow, and how many total calories they consume.
- Lifestyle and diet are still the crucial variables that are within our power to control. By and large, they will determine how corpulent we become. And right now, we are not doing very well.

Lifestyle

It is obvious from the gross numbers that the modern phenomenon of overweight and obesity, now engulfing slightly more than half of all Americans, is largely a function of our lifestyles—including what we eat, when and how we eat it, the type of work we do, the way we spend our free time, and the cumulative impact of modern technologies and inventions. We are victims of our conveniences, the passive forms of entertainment we seek out in our leisure time, our high-fat diets—in general, our affluent way of life. Compared to today, at the turn of the twentieth century, the average American consumed 10 percent more calories per day, but rates

> *Lifestyle and diet are still the crucial variables that are within our power to control. By and large, they will determine how corpulent we become.*

of obesity were only half as great. At the same time, of course, lacking automobiles, personal computers, televisions, and the like, our great-grandparents were much more physically active.

As a general rule of thumb, each pound of fat that we accumulate on our bodies is worth about 3,500 calories when burned. The day-by-day intake of more energy in the form of food and drink than we are able to expend through work, exercise, or resting metabolism—the rate at which our bodies burn energy when we are simply sitting still—results in the steady accretion of pounds. Not all fat is created equal, and not all people are created equal in the efficiency with which they store excess calories as pounds. But this is the basic equation, and over time, this imbalance becomes obvious on our hips, paunches, thighs, and arms. We join the growing throngs of the overweight and, eventually, the obese.

Diseases and Disorders

Researchers currently believe that no more than 1 to 2 percent of obesity cases are caused directly by genetic or medical diseases or disorders. The catalog of genetic disorders known as OMIM (Online Mendelian Inheritance in Man) lists no fewer than 34 genetic syndromes in which obesity is a notable feature.[10] Illustrating how rare most of these disorders are, one of the most common is Prader-Willi syndrome, found in every 25,000 births. In addition to obesity, other features of Prader-Willi syndrome include underdevelopment of the gonads, small hands and feet, and an average survival of no more than 30 years, due to diabetes or heart disease. Many of these genetically linked obesity syndromes (Biemond, Urban-Rogers-Meyer, Chundley, Wilson-Turner, and others) involve mental retardation.

> Researchers currently believe that no more than 1 to 2 percent of obesity cases are caused directly by genetic or medical diseases or disorders.

The following are three of the genetically medically linked obesity syndromes that are clinically important in otherwise healthy adults, and potentially treatable.

Cushing's syndrome. Most often caused when the adrenal glands (which sit atop the kidneys) overproduce a hormone called cortisol because of messages sent to them by a defective pituitary gland (found at the base of the brain). Symptoms include the development of excess fat in the face, abdomen, and in a so-called "buffalo hump" between the shoulders. This disease can be treated by surgery or medications, depending on how early it is detected. Advanced cases can lead to diabetes and complications such as osteoporosis, making spinal fractures more likely. Cushing's can also be caused by tumors or the long-term use of steroids.

Hypothyroidism. The thyroid is a butterfly-shaped gland found at the base of the neck. It produces a hormone that helps regulate the pace of many bodily activities, including the breakdown of fat tissue. Underproduction of this hormone for any one of a variety of reasons—including changes in hormones secreted by the pituitary or the hypothalamus glands, or changes in the thyroid gland itself—can lead to weight gain and other negative symptoms, including dry skin, lethargy, and constipation. This condition is readily detectable by blood-chemistry tests and can be treated by taking replacement thyroid hormones in pill form.

Polycystic ovary syndrome. A relatively common disorder, found in up to 5 percent of women of childbearing age, this syndrome is marked by unvarying high levels of hormones such as estrogen, which normally rise and fall throughout the menstrual cycle. In addition to obesity, seen in about half of the patients who have polycystic ovary syndrome, it can cause the excess growth of body and facial hair (hirsutism), disrupt the menstrual cycle, and make it difficult to conceive a child. It is treatable with several medications, including the diabetes medicine metformin, low-dosage birth-control pills, and weight reduction.

In addition to catalogued genetic disorders, scientists in many laboratories have been busy for the past decade identifying single genes, as well as combinations of genes, that cause marked degrees of obesity in mice and rats. Most of these genes are known to have direct analogues in humans, even if the understanding of how they are expressed to cause obesity is not as advanced for people as it is for rodents.

Six single-gene mouse models of obesity have been developed to date—the *obese* mouse, *diabetes* mouse, *fat* mouse, *tubby* mouse, *yellow* mouse, and *KK* mouse. In these chunky rodents, a change in one gene—which can be either recessive or dominant—has been proven to directly lead to fat offspring. One of the most exciting lines of research involves genes that are responsible for the manufacture and detection of *leptin*, a chemical secreted by fat cells that appears to play a significant role in signaling the brain that adequate stores of fat are present in the body. When the brain's receptors that ordinarily allow it to detect leptin circulating in the blood are not working properly (as in the *diabetes* mouse), or when leptin itself is not being produced due to a genetic defect (as in the *obese* mouse), these little rodents display gigantic appetites, eating almost nonstop and swelling up like balloons. It is as if the leptin-challenged mice lack a shut-off valve that keeps most of their species in fighting trim.

> One of the most exciting lines of research involves genes that are responsible for the manufacture and detection of leptin, a chemical secreted by fat cells that appears to play a significant role in signaling the brain that adequate stores of fat are present in the body.

The possible implications for humans are obvious, but, unfortunately, initial excitement about the possibility of developing drugs based on leptin has faded as researchers' appreciation of the complexities and difficulties of this angle of attack has grown. Hope has not disappeared completely, however. We will review this and other tantalizing lines of research in chapter 8, "On the Horizon."

Disorders of the Hypothalamus

The hypothalamus is an area of the brain that is a central gatekeeper for the body's endocrine, or hormonal, system as well as the autonomic nervous system. It has an important role to play in mood, appetite, and the regulation of basic body processes such as sleep and body temperature. Diseases of the hypothalamus, or its injury from trauma or surgery, can result in a condition known as hypothalamic obesity. This may be due to changes in the secretion of a chemical known as neuropeptide Y, which stimulates eating. In the laboratory, administering neuropeptide Y to test animals provokes overeating. As with leptin, this series of observations has led to many ideas for possible anti-obesity designer drugs, which we will discuss later.

Smoking Cessation

The association between smoking and weight is well known. Tragically, there is evidence that some teenage girls and women smoke because they believe it will help them stay thin—a deadly form of homage to society's cover-girl stereotyping. Indeed, nicotine *is* an appetite suppressant. In addition, smoking can cause an increase of about 10 percent in the body's metabolic rate, which means a smoker literally burns more energy. When a habitual smoker stops smoking, he or she typically experiences weight gain. Studies show that this weight gain averages about 6 to 10 pounds, although there are some people who gain much more. A 1995 study published in the *New England Journal of Medicine* found that during the decade of the 1980s, about one-fourth of the weight gain in male Americans, and one-sixth of the weight gain in female Americans, could be attributed to their successful efforts to stop smoking during that period.[11] Given the known hazards of smoking, it is, perhaps, unnecessary to say that notwithstanding this effect, cigarettes are not recommended for weight control by any health professionals.

Alcohol Consumption

In moderate amounts (no more than the equivalent of one or two ordinary glasses of wine per day), alcohol has not been shown to lead to weight gain—it is a micronutrient-free source of "empty calories."

However, drinking alcohol can be damaging if its use leads to overeating, especially of fats, and even moderate drinking over a prolonged period can be associated with alcoholic fatty liver in individuals who have abdominal obesity. More-than-moderate consumption almost invariably will eventually lead to often deadly and insidious alcoholic liver disease.

Medications Taken for Other Diseases or Disorders

Almost all drugs, no matter how beneficial, have at least some unwanted side effects. Unfortunately, certain members of several important classes of medications can lead to weight gain.

Antidepressants and antimanics. Used in the treatment of mood disorders.

Anti-epileptics. Used to prevent or treat seizures.

Antihypertensives. Used to control high blood pressure.

Phenothiazines. Used in the treatment of schizo-affective disorders (schizophrenia).

Steroids and other hormones. Used for controlling diseases associated with inflammation, such as asthma or inflammatory bowel disease, or for hormonal conditions.

CONDITIONS ASSOCIATED WITH OBESITY

In chapter 2, "Diagnosis: Getting Some Answers," we will talk about the difference between overweight and obesity, and give you some easy ways to determine whether you're in the normal range, the overweight range, or the obese range. Before we get to that, it is important to acknowledge an obvious fact—it is not as damaging to be slightly overweight as it is to be grossly obese.

The list of possible diseases and conditions resulting from overweight and obesity reflects what can go wrong at the upper ranges of obesity, in particular. Most people can weigh up to 20 percent over their ideal body weight without suffering from an excess of diseases. However, just a few extra pounds can have traceable effects.

The closer we get to serious degrees of obesity, though, the worse the effects on many of our vital systems. That's true for each of us individually, and for all of us collectively, as a nation and world. Studies have repeatedly shown that obesity is a risk factor for some of the most debilitating diseases we face. That means that if you are obese, you are at significantly greater risk for developing type 2 diabetes, coronary heart disease, hypertension (high blood pressure), gallbladder disease, osteoarthritis, and a number of different types of cancer. According to the U.S. Centers for Disease Control and Prevention (CDC), overweight and physical inactivity—which usually go hand-in-hand with excess body fat—are responsible for about 300,000 premature deaths annually in the United States. The CDC says that is second only to the number of premature deaths caused by smoking tobacco.

> It is important to acknowledge an obvious fact—it is not as damaging to be slightly overweight as it is to be grossly obese.

Worldwide, the World Health Organization says there are now about 300 million obese adults. It has coined the term *globesity* to describe what it calls "an escalating global epidemic of overweight and obesity." This epidemic is giving health professionals pause both because of its disease impact and because of its enormous price tag—something that may yet gain the attention of both the nation's consumers and its employers, who foot most of the bill for health insurance.

Table 1 provides a summary of something we don't often think about—obesity's economic impact.

Adding up dollars to reach this huge total is one way of driving home the toll that obesity and overweight take on our society. Thinking of it in terms of money may seem a little unemotional, but obesity

Table 1. Medical Conditions Associated with Obesity (and Their Estimated Costs)

Condition	Direct Costs (Related to Overweight and Obesity)[a]	Indirect Costs (Related to Overweight and Obesity)[b]	Total Costs (Related to Overweight and Obesity)
Overweight and Obesity	$51.6 billion (5.7% of total U.S. health expenditures)	$47.6 billion (comparable to total costs of cigarette smoking)	$99.2 billion
Heart Disease	$6.99 billion	—	$6.99 billion
Type 2 Diabetes	$32.4 billion	$30.74 billion	$63.14 billion
Osteoarthritis	$4.3 billion	$12.9 billion	$17.2 billion
Hypertension (High Blood Pressure)	$3.23 billion	—	$3.23 billion
Breast Cancer (Postmenopausal)	$840 million	$1.48 billion	$2.32 billion
Endometrial Cancer	$286 million	$504 million	$790 million
Colon Cancer	$1.01 billion	$1.78 billion	$2.78 billion

Source: Adapted from "Statistics Related to Overweight and Obesity," published on the National Institute of Diabetes and Digestive and Kidney Diseases Web site (www.niddk.nih.gov/health/nutrit/pubs/statobes.htm). Statistics based on 1995 dollars and originally developed by Wolf and Colditz, *Obes Res.* 1998, 6(2): 97–106.

Notes: a. Costs of prevention, diagnosis, and treatment, including all doctor visits, hospital admissions, and medications.
b. Wages lost by people who cannot work due to the condition in question, as well as estimated value of their future earnings, which are not realized due to premature death.

is an issue that hits many in the pocketbook—whether they are shelling out more money for health insurance premiums and copayments, or trying to cope with wages and salary lost due to their own obesity-related diseases or that of their family's breadwinner.

Now let's look at these diseases and conditions from a medical standpoint.

Type 2 Diabetes

Also known as non-insulin-dependent diabetes, this illness is characterized by the body's increasing resistance to the vitally needed action of insulin. Insulin is a hormone, manufactured by the pancreas, which the body needs to transport glucose, or blood sugar, into muscle and other types of cells where it serves as the body's chief form of energy.

With glucose levels rising over time, an overworked pancreas races to produce more insulin, to little effect. Finally, insulin production begins to fall. The symptoms of type 2 diabetes develop more slowly but are, in the end, very similar to those of type 1 diabetes (where the pancreas no longer manufactures insulin at all due to an autoimmune disorder). Consequences can include severe damage to small blood vessels in the eyes, kidneys, and limbs (especially the feet), sometimes leading to the need for amputation. It is believed there are 14 to 15 million people in the United States with type 2 diabetes and that one-third or more of them are not being treated because they have never been diagnosed.

Type 2 diabetes and obesity are very closely related. The disease is almost never found in people with low body fat; about 80 percent of cases occur in the overweight. Driving home that link, the Centers for Disease Control and Prevention reported that cases of diabetes shot up by 33 percent among American adults during the 1990s, during the

> *Thinking of obesity and overweight in terms of money may seem a little unemotional, but obesity is an issue that hits many in the pocketbook—whether they are shelling out more money for health insurance premiums and copayments, or trying to cope with wages and salary lost due to their own obesity-related diseases or that of their family's breadwinner.*

> **Diet and Exercise Attack Diabetes**
>
> One of the most feared medical complications of obesity—and one of the most challenging illnesses anyone can suffer—is type 2 diabetes. The statistical association between obesity and diabetes is extremely strong, as we have discussed. However, since the summer of 2001, there has been dramatic proof that people at risk of diabetes can fight back.
>
> Health and Human Services Secretary Tommy G. Thompson announced that researchers had halted a major study a year earlier than planned because the results were already overwhelmingly clear: Diet and exercise are even more effective than the leading drug in preventing the development of type 2 diabetes.
>
> Researchers studied 3,234 people with impaired glucose tolerance—a condition that often leads to diabetes. Their average Body Mass Index (Body Mass Index will be discussed in chapter 2) was 34, putting them well into the obese category. Their ages ranged from 25 to 85 (average age was 51), and nearly half of them—45 percent—were from minority groups at high risk of type 2 diabetes. Participants were assigned randomly to one of three groups; the first agreed to major lifestyle changes (diet and exercise); the second received the drug metformin; and the third received placebo (inert) pills instead of metformin.

same period in which obesity increased by nearly 60 percent. Moreover, the CDC noted, further "dramatic increases" in diabetes as well as cardiovascular disease can be expected in the future, tracking the underlying bulge in the nation's midsection.

Heart Disease

Excess fatty tissue requires the heart to work harder to circulate the body's blood. The incidence of cardiac arrhythmia (irregular heartbeat), the risk of sudden cardiac death, and the risk of congestive heart

> Although the groups receiving metformin and the placebo pills also received counseling about diet and exercise, the lifestyle change group did more—they engaged in 30 minutes of moderate exercise a day and were also trained to eat a low-fat diet.
>
> In the first year of the study, members of the diet-and-exercise cohort lost an average of 7 percent of their weight, or about 15 pounds, and most of them maintained a 5 percent loss during the 3-year follow-up period.
>
> The heartening results?
>
> Though the group on metformin saw their risk of progressing to diabetes cut nearly by one-third (31 percent), those in the lifestyle-intervention group fared dramatically better. Their risk of progressing to diabetes went down by more than one-half (58 percent).
>
> Over the course of the study, about 29 percent of those on the placebo developed diabetes. About 22 percent of those taking the drug metformin developed diabetes. But only about 14 percent of those on the diet-and-exercise regimen developed diabetes.
>
> Dr. Allen Spiegel, director of the National Institute of Diabetes and Digestive and Kidney Diseases, said the results "represent a major step toward the goal of containing and ultimately reversing the epidemic of type 2 diabetes in this country."[12] If you are obese, losing weight can substantially decrease your risk of developing type 2 diabetes.

failure all increase with obesity, along with the risk of atherosclerosis (coronary artery disease). Growing obesity also contributes to a condition called hyperlipidemia, with heightened levels of dangerous blood fats called LDL cholesterol circulating in the blood, along with lower levels of beneficial blood fats called HDL cholesterol.

Hypertension (High Blood Pressure)

Blood pressure increases with relative body weight. The mechanism for this is not well understood but the effect has been repeatedly observed in large-scale studies for nearly a century. Studies have also shown significant overlap between hypertension, obesity, and diabetes. Hypertension is, in turn, a major risk factor for heart attack, stroke, and kidney damage, including end-stage renal disease, in which kidney failure requires the patient's blood to be filtered through a dialysis machine.

Stroke

Major risk factors for stroke include high blood pressure, diabetes, and heart disease—all of which are known consequences of obesity (see above).

Gallbladder Disease

The body manufactures cholesterol in proportion to the amount of fatty tissue it has. Increases in body fat thus lead to the production of more cholesterol by the liver. Some of this cholesterol gets into the gallbladder fluid and increases its propensity to precipitate into the most common form of gallstones. This can lead, in turn, to chronic inflammation of the gallbladder in some patients. In the Nurses' Health Study, one-third of all cholecystectomies (surgeries to remove the gallbladder) were performed on very overweight or obese women.[13]

Osteoarthritis

Osteoarthritis (OA) is the breakdown in cartilage, the fibrous connective tissue that protects the ends of bones from grinding against each other in a joint. The relationship between obesity and OA is strongest in women and for knee joints, and obesity is the greatest *preventable* risk factor for OA—which is, in turn, the leading overall cause of disability.[14] Obesity may not cause OA directly, but it does hasten OA's progression because of the strain placed on already damaged joints by excess weight.

Sleep Apnea

The buildup of fat in the throat and neck can lead to sleep apnea (interruption of breathing while sleeping), a serious condition that can lead, in turn, to heart failure if not properly treated. Weight loss is the best remedy.

Fatty Liver (Hepatic Steatosis and Nonalcoholic Steatohepatitis)

Both obesity and type 2 diabetes are strongly linked to a form of liver disease that is characterized by excess fat in the liver. In some cases, this can lead to inflammation and progressive liver damage.

Gout

Many studies have demonstrated a link between obesity and gout, a painful disease—often found in the large toe—which is caused when excess uric acid in the blood precipitates into crystals and settles into joints. The growing prevalence of gout may be linked to dietary changes since World War II.

Infertility

Adipose (or fatty) tissue is active biochemically, secreting a powerful form of estrogen called estrone. In obese women, elevated levels of circulating estrogen can interfere with the body's hormonal feedback mechanisms and also result, paradoxically, in higher levels of circulating androgens, or male sex hormones. Disruptions of the menstrual cycle, including failure of the ovaries to release eggs, can follow. Some studies have also shown that the rate of miscarriage is higher in obese women.

Thromboembolism (Blood Clots)

A heightened incidence of blood clots is probably caused by heart disease and poor blood circulation, leading to pooling of blood in the legs. Obese people are at increased risk of blood clots in the veins of the legs, which cause phlebitis, or a clot that lodges in the lungs, which is called a pulmonary embolus.

Cancer

In recent years, there has been a growing recognition of the heightened risks of cancer faced by the obese. In 2001, for the first time, the American Cancer Society (ACS) devoted a special section to obesity in its annual statistical report, highlighting what it called "accumulating evidence" that obesity increases the risk of the following cancers: breast (postmenopausal), uterine, ovarian, and gallbladder cancer in women, and colon and prostate cancer in men.

> *There is accumulating evidence that obesity increases the risk of the following cancers: breast, uterine, ovarian, and gallbladder cancer in women, and colon and prostate cancer in men.*

The ACS stated that the risk of developing breast cancer following menopause is 50 percent higher for obese women; the risk of developing colon cancer is 40 percent higher for obese men; and the risks of developing the more uncommon gallbladder and endometrial (uterine corpus) cancer are 5 times higher for obese people. Further, it went on, there may be a "positive association" between obesity and cancers of the kidney, pancreas, rectum, esophagus, and liver.[15]

Some studies have found that obesity poses a higher risk for colon cancer in women as well as in men, although the effect may be weaker. In June 2001, the World Health Organization released estimates stating that 10 percent of all colon cancers are traceable to obesity, along with 25 percent of all gallbladder cancers.

Dr. Michael Thun, vice president of epidemiology and surveillance research for the ACS, says appreciation of the obesity-cancer connection has been slow developing, in part because the relationship can be complicated. For instance, studies show that obesity may actually reduce a woman's risk of breast cancer prior to menopause, as it can interfere with ovulation. But after menopause, because fatty tissue releases a potent form of estrogen into the blood (as noted earlier), obesity increases a woman's risk of breast cancer. Estrogen is the major promoter of growth in breast cancer. (For the same reason, postmenopausal women and their doctors must weigh the many potential benefits of estrogen-replacement therapy against the increased risk of breast cancer.) To underline this point, the Nurses' Health Study showed that women who gained more than 20 kilograms (about 44 pounds) between the ages of 18 and midlife doubled their risk of developing breast cancer compared with women who did not gain weight.[16] In addition, one study found that after mastectomy for breast cancer, the risk of recurrence of the cancer was increased in women who subsequently gained weight.

With regard to colorectal and prostate cancers, the characteristic apple-shaped pattern of male abdominal obesity may be especially hazardous, as it has been correlated not only with insulin resistance (as described previously) but also with the manufacture of non-insulin growth factors, says Dr. Thun. As with estrogen in women, those non-insulin growth factors can promote tumor growth and progression.

The nexus between diet, obesity, and cancer is an exceedingly active field of study. A recent paper by a noted researcher suggests that a relationship between estrogen exposure, fat intake, obesity, and food cooking and processing in the typical Western-type diet may help to explain the high recent rates of breast and prostate cancer. Of all mammals, only dogs—which were domesticated and underwent a major dietary shift about 10,000 years ago—share the human risk for cancer in their aging prostates, says Donald S. Coffey, a Johns Hopkins urologist. Our best bet for preventing both breast and prostate cancer, he suggests, is to "return to the original diets under which our ancestors evolved"—those rich in fruits and fresh vegetables.[17]

> *A recent paper by a noted researcher suggests that a relationship between estrogen exposure, fat intake, obesity, and food cooking and processing in the typical Western-type diet may help to explain the high recent rates of breast and prostate cancer.*

Of all the cancers the American Cancer Society tracks, the one that is currently showing the most rapid increase is cancer of the esophagus, says Dr. Thun. And that, too, has a known connection to obesity. Obesity predisposes people to develop the condition known as gastroesophageal reflux disease, in which acid and bile from the stomach are partially regurgitated into the lower esophagus after a meal. Heartburn is one of the most common symptoms. Over time, this can lead to changes in the lining of the esophagus (known as Barrett's esophagus), which are precursors to the development of cancer of the lower portion of the esophagus in the same way in which certain polyps in the colon are precursors to the development of colon cancer. "That has been the cancer with the fastest increase in incidence since the mid-1970s," says Dr. Thun, "particularly in white men in North America and Europe."

Most recently, researchers at Harvard reported more evidence tying yet another cancer—that of the pancreas—to obesity. In analyzing data collected from more than 163,000 individuals enrolled in the Health Professionals Follow-Up Study and the Nurses' Health Study, the researchers found that obesity significantly increased the risk of pancreatic cancer. However, a sedentary lifestyle—obesity's frequent twin—was also a key factor, because remaining physically active helped to *decrease* the risk. (Of some interest, as well, is that the study found a significant increase in risk among tall people.)[18]

> *Being obese increases the risk of death from all causes—and especially from heart disease—by 50 to 100 percent, according to a national panel commissioned by the National Institutes of Health to review the scientific literature on obesity and recommend treatment guidelines.*

Bottom Line

A small degree of overweight is not likely to have severe consequences, but obesity—defined as a Body Mass Index (BMI) of 30 or above (see chapter 2)—can shorten life and increase the risk of a variety of health problems. A BMI of 30 or above equates to a 5-foot-3-inch person weighing 169 pounds or more, for example, or a 6-foot-3-inch person weighing 240 pounds or more. (People who are very fit and who have a relatively high percentage of their weight in muscle mass as opposed to fatty tissue may be exceptions to this general yardstick.) Being obese increases the risk of death from all causes—and especially from heart disease—by 50 to 100 percent, according to a national panel commissioned by the National Institutes of Health to review the scientific literature on obesity and recommend treatment guidelines.[19]

To many of us, such dire warnings may sound a bit alarmist. After all, we've kind of gotten used to that extra padding around the middle.

But in 2001, the RAND Institute, a sober think tank that specializes in crunching numbers, issued an eyebrow-raising report. Based on a 1998 telephone survey of 9,585 American adults, RAND reported that obese people report having more chronic health problems—by their own account—than even lifetime smokers or problem drinkers. And in line with national trends, the survey found that nearly three in five Americans are either overweight (36 percent) or obese (23 percent).[20] This largely self-inflicted problem is not going away.

A HEALTHY RESPECT FOR FAT

As a race of mostly carnivores, we all know what fat is when we see it on a steak or a pork chop—it's that white or clear stuff that seems to taste so good when we tuck a little of it onto our forks along with the meat.

But just what, exactly, is the fat inside of *us* that expands our waistlines, thickens our hips and thighs, and lends heft to our upper arms? Where does that fat come from when we gain weight, and where does it go when we lose weight?

Is it a layer of lardlike gunk that builds up under our skin, like sheets of old wax on the kitchen floor?

Is it something that accumulates inside each of the cells composing the normal organs and muscles in our body and makes each of them larger?

Or is it something else entirely?

If you guessed "something else entirely," you're right!

A Fat Breakdown

In fact, fat is its own unique kind of living tissue, called adipose tissue by physiologists. Adipose cells (adipocytes) are a particular kind of cell, enjoying a status similar to that of muscle cells, nerve cells, bone cells, blood cells, and all the other kinds of living cells that compose our bodies.

And like all the other cells, adipose cells have an important job to do. Historically, they have served as an indispensable tool, storing excess food energy when times were good and releasing it during times of need. Body fat was (and is) a valuable reservoir for expectant mothers as well as for hunters and gatherers living off the land. Problem is, our bodies' wonderful ability to protect us against future want by growing adipose tissue has boomeranged against us in an age of double-deck hamburgers, foot-long hot dogs, and super-size sodas.

We still grow the adipose tissue. We grow it all too well in a time of stupendous plenty, as judged by the frugal standards of our distant ancestors scrambling to survive in the wild. And having grown this fatty tissue, we suffer the consequences of having added what amounts to a massive new biological system within our own frames.

That's because fat tissue has a fascinating secret life. It's not just an inert blob of jelly. It's a *living organ* that takes in and releases energy (that's its primary job), but it also interacts in a complex way with many circulating chemicals in the body, called hormones.

Think of fat as an old-fashioned telephone operator, taking in chemical messages from all over the body and firing off new calls of its own in reply (or in more contemporary terms, as a re-router in a computer network). It has been known for years that fat's primary job is to store food energy in the form of fatty acid molecules called *triglycerides* and to release that energy when it is needed. But to perform even that fundamental task, fat tissue must communicate with the brain chemically.

In recent years, science has gained important new insights into how this complex energy exchange is conducted. Based on observations of obese mice, researchers learned that fat cells produce a hormone called *leptin*. The delivery of leptin to receptors in the brain serves as a signal that the body has adequate supplies of fat and that the mouse does not need to eat so much. It is one critical part of the feedback loops by which the body maintains its proper weight.

In 1995, a researcher at Rockefeller University licensed his discovery of the gene that codes for leptin to a drug manufacturer, Amgen, for the then unheard-of sum of $20 million. Many people assumed that leptin would be the basis for the first successful anti-obesity drug in humans. Skip lunch, take leptin, and trick your brain into believing you just ate a double cheeseburger with fries. You stay skinny, but your brain has the satisfying feeling of fullness. Seven years later, though, the work continues. The picture has turned out to be more complex. For one thing, it turns out that obese people have relatively high circulating levels of leptin already. For another, leptin showed inconsistent results when tested in clinical trials to reduce overweight. And, finally, because the leptin protein would be broken down by stomach acids, it can only be taken by injection, which limits its appeal.

Indeed, if anything, leptin serves to underline the deceptively complicated reality of fat and fatty tissue. Like rust, fat never sleeps. In addition to leptin, fatty tissue also releases a version of estrogen, the female hormone, into the bloodstream. It produces a hormonelike substance called *tumor necrosis factor*, which may help to explain the development of insulin resistance in the obese; it also plays a role in the manufacture of angiotensinogen, which is converted by an enzyme produced by the kidney into a chemical that narrows the blood vessels and increases blood pressure.[21]

Recently, some researchers have begun experimenting with some astonishing uses for fat. They believe that fat cells have the capacity to be used as "stem cells"—the undifferentiated form of tissue from which more specialized cells can be derived for various organs in the body. Researchers from UCLA and the University of Pittsburgh reported that they transformed fat cells removed from by liposuction from human hips and thighs into other types of cells, including muscle, cartilage, and bone.[22] A private company has reported it is working along similar lines and may be ready to apply to the U.S. Food and Drug Administration for clinical trials in three years.

So, for all the frustration that flab around your middle has caused you, you may want to treat it with a certain grudging respect. It's got a few tricks in store for you, along with ample reserves of energy.

> Recently, some researchers have begun experimenting with some astonishing uses for fat. They believe that fat cells have the capacity to be used as "stem cells"—the undifferentiated form of tissue from which more specialized cells can be derived for various organs in the body.

JOANNA'S STORY: AGAINST ALL ODDS

All the cards seemed to be stacked against Joanna Givens. How could anyone lose weight in her position?

She had—and has—a sturdy body type. "I've got a linebacker's shoulders," she says with a laugh. "I'm a big-boned person."

She had a mother who sabotaged her efforts to lose weight (but it took years for her to come to that realization).

She had Cushing's disease—one of the rare medical causes of obesity.

Following successful surgery for Cushing's, which involved the removal of part of her pituitary gland, she was placed on steroids for the rest of her life. But steroids, too, cause weight gain.

Not surprisingly, she developed type 2 diabetes, a disorder that often dogs the severely overweight.

To top it all off, Joanna overeats when she is under stress—something else she learned years too late. She was under a lot of stress.

By age 38, Joanna was closer to the proverbial bowling ball than she was to a linebacker. A compact 5 feet, 3 inches tall, she weighed 314 pounds—close to *double* the point (169 pounds) that defines obesity for her height.

"Life was miserable," she says. "I had 30 pounds of fluid in each leg and I had to wear zippered compression stockings. I couldn't wear closed shoes; I had to wear sandals. My diabetes was out of control. I had always been a walker, even though I had been heavy all my life. But I couldn't walk a short distance any more without having to stop and rest. Not so much because I was out of breath, but because of the pain—in my feet, my legs, and my back.

"I had borderline high blood pressure. My personal hygiene was horrible. I couldn't get into the bathtub without having a problem getting back up. Going to the bathroom was a trip in itself. The world is not fat conscious. You go to a public restroom, and there's only one wide stall—for the handicapped. The rest of them are narrow. That's difficult. Go where there's a waiting room, like a doctor's office, and most of the chairs are narrow. Life was horrible."

Finally, her weight reached the point where she could not sleep because of the pain in her legs and back. Her doctor recommended that she get evaluated for a gastric bypass—a risky operation that is recommended only for the morbidly obese, those whose lives are being shortened by excess fat.

Fortunately for Joanna, even though her insurance company would not pay for a gastric bypass operation, the company did agree to pay for her comprehensive evaluation at a university weight-management center. "I was kind of lucky in that sense," she says, "and I am glad I didn't go through the bypass surgery, because I am losing weight without it."

Today, nine months after being placed on a restricted diet, with weekly meetings of a therapy support group to help her and other patients stay on track, Joanna is down to 210 pounds, and she has 200 in her sights. She even thinks 190 is attainable, as her progress—and optimism—build.

"I feel great," she says. "My diabetes is gone. Yes! I was taking two forms of pills to try to control the diabetes. We had to play around with so many different kinds of medicines and they just weren't working. But now it's gone. My blood pressure is actually a little on the low side."

She took off the zippered stockings months ago. "I don't have the fluid retention at all any more."

Like many overweight people, Joanna had tried many different diets and weight-reduction strategies on her own over the years. None of them worked for any length of time. So what's different about this one?

"They don't just throw a diet at you," Joanna says, talking about the university center. "It's very realistic." Part of the realism comes from evaluating each person individually and evaluating his or her medical history, metabolism, and body type before setting a realistic weight-reduction goal.

"Plus you have the support group, and that's really important," she says, referring to weekly meetings with fellow patients and a counselor.

The support group is what allows her to live with the 900-calorie diet—less than half the average American diet. "Five supplements a day and one low-cal, lowfat, low-carb meal doesn't leave you with a lot of options. You have to be very creative. I'm an artist. I went to art school. My best work is in pencil, but I can also do crafts, and I can make jewelry. It helps to be creative on this diet. I've discovered the secrets of making these supplements palatable, and I share that with the group.

"For the one meal a day that I can cook myself, I use a lot of spices and cooking wines. I make soup with bouillon cubes, and I make the supplement shakes with extract—vanilla, orange, banana, almond. I don't like bland food. Anything to change it and make it palatable."

So what of the future? Joanna is taking things one day at a time—or as she says, "one supplement at a time"—but her outlook is positive and her resolve is firm.

"I came across pictures of me from last summer, and it was like—My God! Was I really that fat? I'll never be able to go back to eating like I did. I really think that remembering what I went through at 314 pounds is going to keep me focused, because I never want to get back to that again."

SUMMARY

Nature bred us for sterner stuff than scurrying around like mall rats. Our distant ancestors burned all the calories they could consume as hunters and gatherers. Walking from the SUV to the supermarket freezer to stash away our next gallon of rocky road doesn't cut it—not even if it's lowfat. Experts differ on whether obesity should be termed a disease or a physical condition, but all agree that a sedentary lifestyle is responsible for the majority of obese people in our society. Genetic diseases and conditions that cause obesity do exist but are not usually the culprit. Sadly, experts also agree that regardless of how it's caused, obesity itself often leads to a host of other diseases and conditions—from gout and gallbladder disease to type 2 diabetes, a serious illness that is skyrocketing as a direct echo of the obesity boom. Evidence also increasingly points to a connection between obesity and several types of cancer. Clearly, being seriously overweight can cost us much more than the price of a new wardrobe.

> *Experts differ on whether obesity should be termed a disease or a physical condition, but all agree that a sedentary lifestyle is responsible for the majority of obese people in our society.*

CHAPTER 2

Diagnosis
Getting Some Answers

WHEN IT COMES to the problem of obesity, the words from the comic strip *Pogo*, created by the late Walt Kelly, come to mind: "We have met the enemy, and he is us." Given that 61 percent of adult Americans fall into the categories defined as overweight or obese, and with a rapid rise in the rate of obesity among children and youth, there is the danger of painting with too broad a brush. The presence of overweight is all around us—at our kitchen table, in the next cubicle, staring back in the mirror. To make any sense of something so nearly universal, we need to begin to draw distinctions. Common sense tells us that overweight and obesity cannot possibly pose identical risks to each of the three of every five of us who carry around excess baggage. Indeed, they do not. Risks vary by weight, height, body type, metabolism, gender, age, ethnic background, family history, and more—including whether an overweight person has any other medical conditions, such as diabetes.

To understand your specific risks, you would have to undergo the kind of comprehensive evaluation that is performed at the Johns Hopkins Weight Management Center (which will be described later in this chapter). And to calculate your personal vulnerabilities even more precisely, doctors would need the detailed knowledge from your genetic blueprint, as well as a comprehensive understanding of the genetics of obesity in general—which, at this stage of scientific understanding, continues to elude us. A full genetic scan may be part of every medical examination in a couple of decades, but not now. In 2002, and for the foreseeable future, doctors must keep making calculated guesses about who is likely to run into health problems and make treatment recommendations based on this incomplete information.

In essence, some medical recommendations are based on playing the odds—we simply cannot tell who will suffer a heart attack as a result of their excess weight and who will instead die peacefully in their sleep at age 99. That means just about everyone is encouraged to keep their weight down within the recommended limits that have been developed by observing thousands of people in hundreds of studies over the past century.

> *The degree of overweight is important in determining how bad the health effects from the excess fat will be. So is the distribution of fat on the person's body.*

As noted earlier, the *degree* of overweight is important in determining how bad the health effects from the excess fat will be. So is the *distribution* of fat on the person's body. A pear shape—with fat worn mostly around the hips, buttocks, and thighs—is not as bad for the heart, for instance, as is an apple shape with bulging waistline (see figure 2.1). Thus overweight women—who are usually pear-shaped as opposed to apple-shaped—tend on average to face a different pattern of health risks than men. This, in addition to the protective effects of female sex hormones, may be the most important reason that the risk of heart disease does not usually appear even in overweight women until after menopause.

In addition, many health issues hinge on the question of where obesity appears in the life span. Overweight that begins in infancy or childhood may be much more problematic over the course of a lifetime than the type of overweight that presents itself as "middle-aged spread" (see chapter 7, "Family, Society, and Our Overweight Kids").

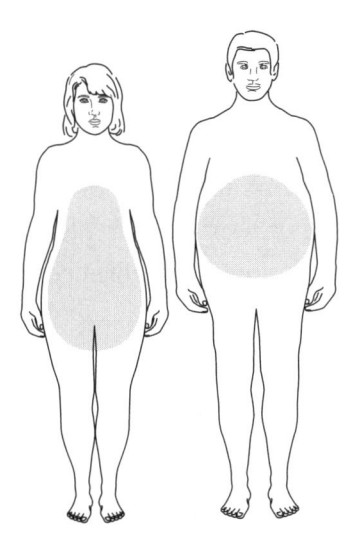

Figure 2.1—*"Apple-" and "Pear-"Shaped Distributions of Fat*

So what's healthy, what's not, and how can you distinguish between the two?

SYMPTOMS AND SIGNS

Medical doctors distinguish between *symptoms* (things that a patient feels or experiences) and *signs* (things a doctor observes). The following are some common signs and symptoms of obesity:

Symptoms. Inability to perform routine activities of life or work with your normal ease (for instance, it becomes difficult to bend over to tie your shoes; to get in and out of the bathtub easily; to climb short flights of stairs or to go on short walks). Other symptoms include increasing shortness of breath (known medically by the term *dyspnea*). You may have an increasing sensation of fatigue with normal exertion. Gastroesophageal reflex or "heartburn" may bother you after meals or at bedtime. You may encounter increasing sleep difficulties.

Signs. Excess body fat as measured through a variety of techniques to be described shortly. Hypertension (high blood pressure). Striae (stretch marks) from cycles of weight loss and gain. Blood tests or urine that reveal a high glucose level (signs of diabetes mellitus).

It is important to note that obesity is only one of the causes of these symptoms and signs; for example, shortness of breath could also be a symptom of chronic lung or heart disease. Please consult with a healthcare professional if you develop an unexplained symptom or sign.

DEFINING OVERWEIGHT AND OBESITY

You can be overweight without being obese. Obesity is a degree of overweight that surpasses a certain cutoff level. The very word *overweight* implies that everyone has a normal, or healthy, weight that is possible to determine. And indeed, doctors believe that this is so.

> *You can be overweight without being obese. Obesity is a degree of overweight that surpasses a certain cutoff level.*

Ideal Body Weight

You may have heard the phrase *ideal body weight* (IBW). Ideal body weight was originally defined as the weight associated with the lowest risk of death (relative to a person's height and gender) among those who purchased life insurance from the Metropolitan Life Insurance Company. Over the course of the 20th century, the concept evolved as physicians and dietitians gradually reached consensus on healthy-weight guidelines. Generally speaking, most people's IBW will fall within ranges that are determined by height. However, a person's specific IBW is highly individual. The following are some of the factors that go into determining the IBW.

Sex. At any given height, men—on average—have a higher IBW than women. That's because men tend to have—on average—greater bone mass and more muscle than women.

Muscularity. At any given height, someone who is physically fit—especially someone who has developed his or her muscle tone—will have a higher IBW than someone who is out of shape. A given volume of muscle (often referred to as *lean muscle mass*) weighs more than a given volume of body fat.

Body build. Some people are simply built larger than others because of their underlying bone structure. At any given height, they will have a higher IBW than someone who inherited a slender build. Researchers conventionally divide body types into three categories—small, medium, and large—according to an odd unit of measure, the width of the elbow, which has been found to be a good marker for the size of the underlying skeleton.

Pregnancy. Weight gain is natural and healthy at the time of pregnancy. However, recommendations for how much weight an expectant mother should gain will vary depending on her size prior to conception. Some doctors say that women in the normal weight range may gain 25 to 35 pounds but that those who are already overweight going into their pregnancies should gain no more than 25. Many women report that pregnancies are "trigger events" that catapult them into obesity and that their base weight increases from pregnancy to pregnancy. Some studies have found average long-term weight gain from each pregnancy to be 9 pounds.[1] It is believed that breast-feeding may release hormones that work against weight gain. In addition, regular exercise is important for the new mother following childbirth, although the pressures of home and children may make it difficult.

Age. The special issue of obesity in children and youth will be addressed in chapter 7. On the other end of the aging spectrum, healthy women and men typically begin gaining body fat—and gradually losing lean muscle mass—in middle age. Men appear to gain body fat at the rate of 2 to 3 percent per decade and women at the rate of 4 to 5 percent per decade between the ages of 40 and 81. It is also common for women to gain weight at the onset of menopause, along with increases in waist size, upper body fat, and lipoproteins (blood fats)—all of which are risk factors for coronary artery disease. However, adjusted healthy-weight standards have not been developed yet for seniors.

Some experts believe they should be judged by the same standards that apply to younger adults, whereas others believe the guidelines, like comfortable belts, should be eased out a notch for the old. Experts do agree that obesity in older adults poses all the same health risks that it does in younger people. They also agree that exercise for seniors, including weight-resistance training, is extremely beneficial in promoting lean muscle mass and fighting overweight. As in younger adults, extra baggage around the waist is especially risky.

> *The good news is that you can get a pretty good handle on your own healthy weight before you ever spend the first dollar on a doctor visit.*

By now, it's probably clear that determining your particular IBW with any degree of precision is, in the end, a job for a health professional devoted to weight management. But the good news is that you can get a pretty good handle on your own healthy weight before you ever spend the first dollar on a doctor visit. Here's how.

First, if you know your height and weight, look at table 2, which is based on recommendations adopted by the National Research Council of the National Academy of Sciences.

Thus, if you're 5 feet, 5 inches tall and 140 pounds, say, or 6 feet, 5 inches and 200 pounds, you pass the first test. You're comfortably within the range of healthy weight. But bear in mind these are averages only. If you're badly out of shape, you may be packing a lot of fat instead of muscle. Also, the above ranges are rather wide because they apply jointly to men and women.

If you are "off the charts" of the healthy-weight range for your height, or if you are in the upper end of your range, you may want to know more about how overweight you are. That's easy to determine, too. But first, let's be a little more precise about what we mean by these terms *overweight* and *obesity*.

Overweight is weighing more than your IBW to such a degree that you are at risk of developing some of the associated medical conditions we have talked about earlier, including type 2 diabetes, high blood pressure, or heart disease.

Table 2. Healthy Weight Ranges for Men and Women

Height (feet and inches, barefoot)	Weight (pounds, unclothed)
5'0"	97–128
5'1"	101–132
5'2"	104–137
5'3"	107–141
5'4"	111–146
5'5"	114–150
5'6"	118–155
5'7"	121–160
5'8"	125–164
5'9"	129–169
5'10"	132–174
5'11"	136–179
6'0"	140–184
6'1"	144–189
6'2"	148–195
6'3"	152–200
6'4"	156–205
6'5"	160–211
6'6"	164–216

Source: Adapted from Lawrence J. Cheskin, *Losing Weight for Good* (Baltimore: Johns Hopkins Univ. Press, 1997).

Obesity is when your degree of overweight becomes pronounced enough that you are at significant risk for a shortened life expectancy. In other terms, obesity is sometimes defined as weighing 30 percent or more above your IBW. Thus if you are 5 feet, 5 inches and your IBW is 140, 30 percent of that weight would be 42 pounds. If you tip the scales at 182 or more (42 pounds above your IBW), you would be considered obese by this rule of thumb. But this is based on the concept of your ideal weight, which is very individual and impossible to determine from a chart. Therefore, researchers have developed another standard—the Body Mass Index—which treats the categories of healthy weight, overweight, and obesity in terms of *ranges* of weight for each height. For more on that, read on.

Extreme obesity (also called *morbid obesity*) is when your obesity is so great that it poses an imminent threat of shortening your life. We will provide you with a chart in the following section that will clarify if you are at risk of falling into this category, which is the point where doctors begin considering such severe alternatives as gastric bypass surgery. One study of young men who were 100 percent or more overweight (i.e., double their healthy weight) found that they had a death rate 12 times higher than men of normal weight.[2] Aside from the risk of premature death, extremely obese individuals are more likely to be very limited in their physical mobility and activities, and to have major health problems. Unfortunately, this is the fastest-growing segment of obese individuals. The percentage of the population comprised of those individuals falling into the dangerously obese category has actually doubled in the past 15 years.

> *The percentage of the population comprised of those individuals falling into the dangerously obese category has actually doubled in the past 15 years.*

Body Mass Index

By international consensus—developed by experts advising such bodies as the World Health Organization and the National Institutes of

Health—there is an actual mathematical formula that can be used to determine your degree of overweight or obesity. As mentioned earlier, it is called the *Body Mass Index (BMI)*.

Because it is an international formula, the BMI is expressed in terms of *kilograms* for weight and *meters* for height. To calculate someone's BMI you divide their weight in kilograms by their height in meters squared.

$$\text{BMI} = \frac{\text{weight in kilograms}}{\text{height in meters} \times \text{height in meters}}$$

As you may not know the metric measures for your height and weight, this formula can be modified to work with pounds and inches by simply multiplying your result by 705.

$$\text{BMI} = \frac{\text{weight in pounds}}{\text{height in inches} \times \text{height in inches}} \times 705$$

So, for example, say that you are 5 feet 6 inches (66 inches) and you weigh 200 pounds. Your weight in pounds (200) divided by 66 inches squared (4,356) is 0.0459. Multiply that by 705 and you get 32.37. If that's your BMI, it's not a good number, as you will see shortly.

Not that much of a mathematician? You'd want to have a calculator available for tackling this one, for sure. An easier way to find your BMI is to consult the Body Mass Index Chart from the National Heart, Lung, and Blood Institute (see table 3). Locate your height (without shoes) in inches on the left, and read across until you find the number corresponding to your weight (unclothed) in pounds. Then follow that column up to the top to find your BMI.

You may note that the formula for BMI pays no attention to whether you are a man or a woman, 20 years old or 70 years old, a marathon

> *You may note that the formula for BMI pays no attention to whether you are a man or a woman, 20 years old or 70 years old, a marathon runner or a couch potato. In other words, like all the other measures we have discussed so far, it is a general set of guidelines that gives doctors a place to start in evaluating any particular individual.*

Table 3. Body Mass Index Chart

BMI	19	20	21	22	23	24	25	26	27	28	29	30	31	32	33	34	35	36
Height (inches)									Body Weight (pounds)									
58	91	96	100	105	110	115	119	124	129	134	138	143	148	153	158	162	167	172
59	94	99	104	109	114	119	124	128	133	138	143	148	153	158	163	168	173	178
60	97	102	107	112	118	123	128	133	138	143	148	153	158	163	168	174	179	184
61	100	106	111	116	122	127	132	137	143	148	153	158	164	169	174	180	185	190
62	104	109	115	120	126	131	136	142	147	153	158	164	169	175	180	186	191	196
63	107	113	118	124	130	135	141	146	152	158	163	169	175	180	186	191	197	203
64	110	116	122	128	134	140	145	151	157	163	169	174	180	186	192	197	204	209
65	114	120	126	132	138	144	150	156	162	168	174	180	186	192	198	204	210	216
66	118	124	130	136	142	148	155	161	167	173	179	186	192	198	204	210	216	223
67	121	127	134	140	146	153	159	166	172	178	185	191	198	204	211	217	223	230
68	125	131	138	144	151	158	164	171	177	184	190	197	203	210	216	223	230	236
69	128	135	142	149	155	162	169	176	182	189	196	203	209	216	223	230	236	243
70	132	139	146	153	160	167	174	181	188	195	202	209	216	222	229	236	243	250
71	136	143	150	157	165	172	179	186	193	200	208	215	222	229	236	243	250	257
72	140	147	154	162	169	177	184	191	199	206	213	221	228	235	242	250	258	265
73	144	151	159	166	174	182	189	197	204	212	219	227	235	242	250	257	265	272
74	148	155	163	171	179	186	194	202	210	218	225	233	241	249	256	264	272	280
75	152	160	168	176	184	192	200	208	216	224	232	240	248	256	264	272	279	287
76	156	164	172	180	189	197	205	213	221	230	238	246	254	263	271	279	287	295

Source: National Heart, Lung, and Blood Institute (www.nhlbi.nih.gov/health/public/heart/obesity/lose_wt/bmi_dis.htm).

runner or a couch potato. In other words, like all the other measures we have discussed so far, it is a general set of guidelines that gives doctors a place to start in evaluating any particular individual. These guidelines were developed for adults age 20 or over and may not apply well to unusually muscular individuals. You can find BMI charts for children and teens in chapter 7.

Now that you have an understanding of what is meant by BMI, let's take another look at stages of overweight in terms of the following internationally accepted standard:

Underweight means having a BMI of less than 18.5. To be this underweight carries medical risks of its own, whether you are a young adult suffering from anorexia or a senior who is undernourished.

Healthy weight means having a BMI of 18.5 to 24.9.

BMI	37	38	39	40	41	42	43	44	45	46	47	48	49	50	51	52	53	54
Height (inches)							Body Weight (pounds)											
58	177	181	186	191	196	201	205	210	215	220	224	229	234	239	244	248	253	258
59	183	188	193	198	203	208	212	217	222	227	232	237	242	247	252	257	262	267
60	189	194	199	204	209	215	220	225	230	235	240	245	250	255	261	266	271	276
61	195	201	206	211	217	222	227	232	238	243	248	254	259	264	269	275	280	285
62	202	207	213	218	224	229	235	240	246	251	256	262	267	273	278	284	289	295
63	208	214	220	225	231	237	242	248	254	259	265	270	278	282	287	293	299	304
64	215	221	227	232	238	244	250	256	262	267	273	279	285	291	296	302	308	314
65	222	228	234	240	246	252	258	264	270	276	282	288	294	300	306	312	318	324
66	229	235	241	247	253	260	266	272	278	284	291	297	303	309	315	322	328	334
67	236	242	249	255	261	268	274	280	287	293	299	306	312	319	325	331	338	344
68	243	249	256	262	269	276	282	289	295	302	308	315	322	328	335	341	348	354
69	250	257	263	270	277	284	291	297	304	311	318	324	331	338	345	351	358	365
70	257	264	271	278	285	292	299	306	313	320	327	334	341	348	355	362	369	376
71	265	272	279	286	293	301	308	315	322	329	338	343	351	358	365	372	379	386
72	272	279	287	294	302	309	316	324	331	338	346	353	361	368	375	383	390	397
73	280	288	295	302	310	318	325	333	340	348	355	363	371	378	386	393	401	408
74	287	295	303	311	319	326	334	342	350	358	365	373	381	389	396	404	412	420
75	295	303	311	319	327	335	343	351	359	367	375	383	391	399	407	415	423	431
76	304	312	320	328	336	344	353	361	369	377	385	394	402	410	418	426	435	443

Overweight is defined as having a BMI of 25 to 29.9.

Obesity is defined as having a BMI of 30 or above.

Extreme (or morbid) obesity is defined as having a BMI of 40 or above.

Waist Circumference

There is one other gender-specific measure that doctors consider very important in determining your degree of overweight. Indeed, some think it is so telltale that it can be considered an alarm bell in its own right, independent of the overall BMI. That is *waist circumference*, which provides a fairly direct measurement of abdominal fat—the worst kind you can be carrying. Anybody who's shopped recently for clothes probably knows his or her waist measurement. Many researchers agree that independent of everything else, women who have waist measurements of more than 35 inches are at risk for obesity-associated conditions, whereas men who have waist measurements of more than 40 inches are at risk.

To measure your waist circumference, take a measuring tape and place it just above the top of your right hipbone (iliac crest, see figure 2.2). Wrap it all the way around your abdomen at that level, being careful to stay horizontal. The tape should not be drawn so tightly as to compress your skin. You should let your breath out to the degree you normally do when breathing.

Armed with the knowledge of your BMI and your waist circumference, you can now get some real inside knowledge about yourself and your particular set of medical risks. Bear in

> *Armed with the knowledge of your BMI and your waist circumference, you can now get some real inside knowledge about yourself and your particular set of medical risks.*

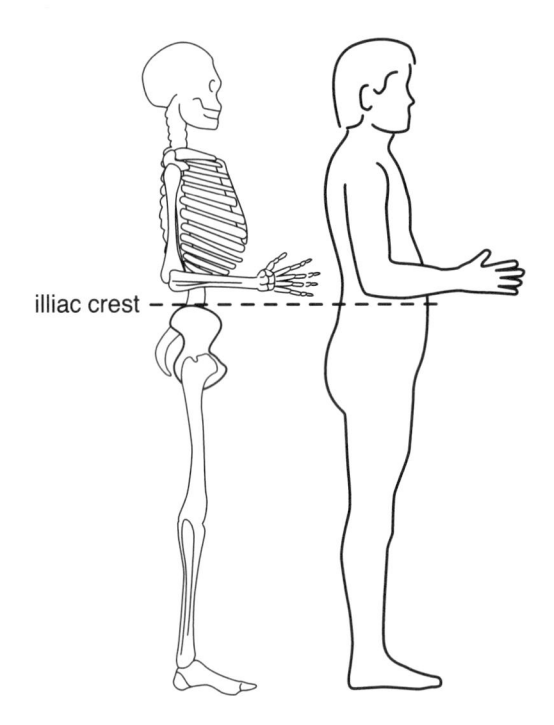

Figure 2.2—*Measuring Waist Circumference*

mind this will not substitute for a doctor visit. However, it may give you added impetus to make an appointment for yourself!

Table 4 allows you to perform a quick self-assessment of your medical risk for type 2 diabetes, high blood pressure, and heart disease relative to people of normal BMI and waist measure. Thus for instance, if you are a woman whose waist measures 36 inches or more and whose BMI is 40 or more, you are considered to be at "extremely high" relative risk of developing these medical complications. If you are a man whose waist measures 40 inches or more and whose BMI is 40 or more, you are in the same boat.

Table 4. Classification of Overweight and Obesity by BMI, Waist Circumference, and Associated Disease Risks

	BMI	Obesity Class	Disease Risk[a] Relative to Normal Weight and Waist	
			Men (40 inches or less) *Women (35 inches or less)*	*Men (More than 40 inches)* *Women (More than 35 inches)*
Underweight	<18.5		-	-
Normal	18.5–24.9		-	-[b]
Overweight	25.0–29.9		Increased	High
Obesity	30.0–34.9	I	High	Very High
	35.0–39.9	II	Very High	Very High
Extreme Obesity	40.0+	III	Extremely High	Extremely High

Source: Adapted from National Heart, Lung, and Blood Institute Web site (*www.nhlbi.nih.gov/health/public/heart/obesity/lose_wt/bmi_dis.htm*).

Notes: a. Disease risk for type 2 diabetes, hypertension, and cardiovascular disease.
      b. Increased waist circumference can be a marker for increased risk even in people of normal weight.

MEASURING BODY FAT

Again, all of the above charts and measures are only averages. To understand your personal situation and its health implications, you should be evaluated by a medical doctor, preferably at a comprehensive weight-management clinic. Doctors who specialize in weight management have a variety of means to assess the amount of body fat you are carrying and the degree to which it is unhealthy for you. For many purposes, your BMI and waist circumference may be all you and your doctor need to evaluate your degree of obesity in order to devise a personal weight-reduction goal and treatment plan, and to track your progress toward that goal. However, if there is doubt about whether you are obese—or about its magnitude—your doctor may want to perform one of several tests to measure your body fat directly.

> *To understand your personal situation and its health implications, you should be evaluated by a medical doctor, preferably at a comprehensive weight-management clinic.*

Tests for Body Fat

As we have noted previously, not all fat is created equal. For instance, excess fat located on the abdomen and upper body has been well established to pose a greater risk for heart disease than excess fat on the hips and thighs. And, healthy-weight ranges, though statistically well founded, may need to be modified for specific individuals because of unusual muscularity or fitness, a very slight or stocky body build, or other reasons. Healthy-weight ranges also do not apply very well to adults who are under 5 feet tall. Therefore, a number of other techniques have been devised for the individualized assessment of body fat.

Skinfold caliper. At one time, many doctors relied on what is colloquially known as the "pinch test," using a plierslike instrument called a *skinfold caliper* to determine the amount of excess body fat as well as its distribution on the body. This test is no longer widely used but you may still run into it. In 2001, a professor of epidemiology at the University of Minnesota found that so many people are so overweight that the pinch test is no longer statistically valid. About one-fourth of 50-year-old women are so overweight that the skin folds on the backs of their thighs, backs of their arms, and on their backs and waists are too thick to be measured reliably.[3]

Bioelectrical impedance. Coming into wider use is the *bioelectrical impedance test*, which measures the *total body electrical conductivity*. A small instrument that somewhat resembles a bathroom scale is used to run a very weak electrical current through the body. The test is painless. Because fat tissue does not conduct electricity as well as muscle mass, this device provides a measure of the overall percentage of body fat. However, it may not be dependable in cases of extreme obesity. So-called "body fat analyzers" are being widely sold as consumer items. Although the scientific principle behind these products is valid, most doctors would say there is no reason to spend your dollars this way. Your BMI and waist-circumference measures, which you may obtain for free, usually provide all the information that is needed to evaluate your degree of overweight and devise an appropriate plan. Medical doctors often use bioimpedance as an adjunct to the BMI to see whether people who have lost weight are preserving their lean muscle mass (losing fat rather than muscle.) In other words, if you fail to exercise and do strength training, you could lose weight and have a better BMI, but not be less "fatty" as a proportion of your total weight.

Total body water. Don't try this at home! Some weight-management clinics might weigh you while you are immersed in a tank of water and compare that number with your weight on dry land. Because fat tissue is not as dense as lean muscle mass (scientists say it has a lower *specific gravity*), the comparison of the two weights gives a good measure of your percentage of body fat.

Imaging. *Imaging* tests that a doctor may use to get more detailed information about the precise size and location of fat deposits on your body include:

- CT (computed tomography)
- MRI (magnetic resonance imaging)
- Dual-energy x ray absorptiometry

As their names might imply, these tests all involve radiation. CT uses x rays to obtain very detailed cross-sectional views of your entire body. MRI uses non-ionizing radiation (akin to radio waves) to image your body. Dual-energy x ray absorptiometry uses low doses of x rays to measure differences in the density of soft tissues and bones. Although none of these tests poses a high degree of risk, they are all relatively expensive and depend on sophisticated equipment. Doctors will likely order these tests only if they are concerned about specific medical conditions that might be associated with your overweight.

WHO IS AT RISK?

The United States, and much of the rest of the world, has grown steadily more obese in the past half-century. But Americans really ballooned in the 1990s. Increases in our national girth were observed across the board. Based on annual nationwide surveys, the Centers for Disease Control and Prevention reports that obesity (defined as a BMI of 30 or above) shot up from 12 percent in 1991 to 18.9 percent in 1999—an increase of nearly 60 percent in less than a decade![4]

A couple of trends within the totals stood out:

- Obesity among thirtysomethings rose by 10 percent in just one year, from 1998 to 1999. (A separate study found the incidence of diabetes in this age group increased by 70 percent in the 1990s.)
- The largest *increase* in obesity from 1998 to 1999 occurred among whites, at 7 percent. But overall, blacks were showing the highest *percentage* of obesity (27.3 percent), followed by Hispanics (21.5 percent), whites (17.7 percent), and all others (12.4 percent).

Researchers know there are a few persistent factors that point to special risks of becoming obese. One predictor is socioeconomic status. Obesity is more prevalent in lower-income groups (although recent data show the rate of obesity is now increasing faster among those who have had some college education than among those who have only high school). As long ago as the 1960s, researchers reported that overweight was nine times as common in the lowest-income groups they studied (36 percent) as it was in the highest-income groups (4 percent).[5] This was even more true for women than it was for men. Various theories have been advanced to explain this difference, including unequal access to the best-quality health care, unequal access to the healthiest foods, unequal access to education, and the force of peer pressure operating on the affluent to remain slender.

> *Researchers know there are a few persistent factors that point to special risks of becoming obese.*

In addition, anyone who has stopped smoking, or is getting ready to stop smoking, is at risk of weight gain, 6 to 10 pounds on average, but sometimes much more. This common situation poses a host of special considerations. Given smokers' high lifetime risks for emphysema, lung cancer, and heart disease, among other medical conditions, smoking cessation is definitely recommended. But trading a pack a day for obesity is not always a good swap—nor is it necessary (see sidebar, "Women Smokers Fear Weight Gain").

A strong family history of obesity is also a strong indicator of personal risk. This, again, is likely true for a combination of genetic, dietary, cultural, and psychological reasons. We will try to unravel the complex threads of psychology, self-image, and learned behavior as they relate to obesity in chapter 7.

MEDICAL EVALUATION

If you've read this far, odds are good that you have flunked some of the tests we've discussed. Maybe your BMI is well into the range

Women Smokers Fear Weight Gain

For years, tobacco companies have understood the connection in many women's minds between smoking and thinness and have played to it with cunningly merchandised smokes such as Virginia Slims.

That association is so indelible that fear of gaining weight is one of the principal reasons why women, in general, find it harder to quit smoking than men do, say researchers. "It would be an important clinical advance if we find a way to successfully address those concerns, making it easier for more women to stop smoking," says Dr. Alan Leshner, director of the National Institute on Drug Abuse.[6]

In a telltale study published in the August 2001 issue of *Journal of Consulting and Clinical Psychology,* researchers at the University of Pittsburgh School of Medicine recruited 219 women smokers who wanted to quit but who voiced fears about gaining weight after they gave up cigarettes. The women were divided into three groups: one that received standard smoking-cessation therapy; one that received standard smoking-cessation therapy plus dietary advice; and one that received standard smoking-cessation therapy plus additional counsel-

---

above 30. Maybe you were stunned at how much of the tape measure you needed to pull out to encircle your waist. Maybe your love handles or thighs haven't passed your own "pinch test" for a couple of years now. Or maybe you have tried and failed, over a period of time, to take off excess fat through a series of short-lived desperation diets, and you are ready for something more comprehensive and systematic—something that can become part of your life.

Not surprisingly, if you are obese and ready to get serious about slimming down, doctors recommend that you begin with comprehensive evaluation by a physician. You could begin by making an appointment with whomever delivers your primary care. This could be either of the following:

ing to address their concerns about weight gain head-on. In essence, women in the last group were advised that gaining weight would be less damaging to their health than continuing to smoke.

At the end of one year, the women in the weight-counseling group—despite having been discouraged from dieting—had actually gained *less* weight than the other two groups, including the group that received dietary advice. They gained an average of 5.5 pounds, as compared to 11.9 and 16.9 pounds in the dietary advice and standard-therapy groups, respectively. Moreover, more of those in the weight-counseling group were able to quit smoking without relapse (21 percent) than those in the dietary-advice and standard-therapy groups (13 percent and 9 percent, respectively).

Researcher Kenneth Perkins thus concludes that "overconcern about weight gain," as opposed to actual weight gain, may be what leads to smoking relapse for many women. Without question, many health professionals would be overjoyed to have this finding confirmed in future studies—that greater realism about weight gain can lead both to lower weight gain *and* to a heightened likelihood of smoking cessation.

Family physician. An M.D. (or, more infrequently, a D.O., or doctor of osteopathy) who sees the entire family for routine medical care, making referrals to specialists or admissions to hospitals as medical needs might dictate. Family physicians are sometimes called general practitioners.

Obstetrician/gynecologist. Many women, particularly in their reproductive years, turn to their obstetricians or gynecologists as their primary-care providers, as they usually see them on an annual basis for Pap tests and other regular checkups.

If you don't have a regular doctor—and unfortunately, many people do not—you can contact your local medical society or a specialty listing, such as the American Board of Internal Medicine's Web site (www.abim.org) to find a board-certified physician; or ask local hospitals for a list of board-certified doctors on their staff who are accepting new patients. Most hospitals are happy to furnish lists of area doctors who are affiliated with them in that they have admitting privileges—that is, they have been approved to check their patients into the hospital as required. If you have health insurance, you probably have been given a list of qualified providers in your plan or network. Whatever the list you have, you might consider looking especially for one of the following:

Internist. Medical doctor who specializes in the study of the body's internal organs, their normal functions, and the diagnosis and treatment of their diseases and disorders.

Deciphering the Code

People seeking professional help for weight problems sometimes find the maze of potential providers to be a little bewildering.

Here's a quick key to some of the most frequently encountered acronyms and credentials:

- M.D.—medical doctor (graduate of accredited medical school, licensed by state)
- N.D.—doctor of naturopathy (practices systems of natural healing that do not involve drugs or surgery; is not licensed and cannot order prescription drugs)
- D.O.—doctor of osteopathy (graduate of accredited osteopathy school, licensed by state; equivalent to M.D. in ability to order prescription drugs)
- D.C.—doctor of chiropractic (specializes in treatment of diseases and disorders through manipulation of the spine; can order some prescription drugs relating to musculoskeletal problems)

Endocrinologist. Medical doctor who has advanced training in the study of the body's glands and hormones. Among other things, endocrinologists specialize in the treatment of diabetes and thyroid disorders, two medical conditions that are frequently associated with obesity.

Gastroenterologist. Medical doctor who specializes in the study and treatment of digestive diseases and disorders. Gastroenterologists are experts in issues involving the esophagus, stomach, intestines, gallbladder, liver, and bile ducts.

Bariatric physician. Doctor who specializes in the treatment of obesity, including the use of medications to control appetite. Bariatric physicians can be either M.D.s or D.O.s. This possibility is mentioned last because the number of bariatric physicians is so small compared to the other medical specialties described above. You can obtain

- D.Pod.—doctor of podiatry (specializes in treating disorders of the feet)
- M.A./M.S./M.S.W.—counselors who have master's degrees in psychology or social work
- Ph.D., Psy.D.—psychologists; may be a doctor of philosophy (Ph.D.) or a doctor of psychology (Psy.D.)
- R.D.—registered dietitian (trained in food and nutrition; has a bachelor's or master's degree, has completed an accredited practice program, and has passed a national examination)
- D.T.R.—dietetic technician, registered (has at least a 2-year associate's degree, has completed a technician program, and has passed a national examination)
- R.C.E.P.—registered clinical exercise physiologist (has a graduate degree in exercise science, exercise physiology, or physiology, and has passed a national exam)

a list of the bariatric physicians in your state from the American Society of Bariatric Physicians Web site (www.asbp.org/locate.htm) or by calling (303) 779-4833.

Doctors highly recommend that you begin the exciting journey to a new, sleeker you with a medical checkup for two compelling reasons. First, your life might be at stake. Self-diagnosis is always dangerous. It may be obvious to you that you are too heavy, and it may be obvious to you that you are showing some of the characteristic symptoms of obesity. However, a thorough medical checkup may find that there is a hidden "X" factor at work. A 56-year-old man once came into the Johns Hopkins Weight Management Center and reported that he became short of breath very quickly when he tried to exercise. This was not unexpected because he was more than 50 pounds overweight. However, through a medical exam, it was discovered that he was *also* suffering from the early stages of congestive heart failure, a condition that could have cost him his life. His heart condition was treated successfully—and he was helped to shed 50 pounds. It turned out that his breathlessness was due more to his heart failure than it was to the excess baggage he was carrying around. Only a careful physical exam can find this kind of masked condition.

The second compelling reason for getting a medical exam is that it may uncover a medical cause for your obesity that is not obvious to you. Two classic examples are hypothyroidism and polycystic ovary syndrome, discussed in chapter 1. You can swallow all the slimming shakes, participate in all the encounter groups, and starve your way through all the holiday dinners and weekend cookouts you want. But if you suffer from hypothyroidism or polycystic ovary syndrome, your body chemistry may sabotage your best efforts. You will find that trying to lose weight will be more than tough sledding. It will be like trying to sled uphill—in July.

The National Institutes of Health recommends that you get a medical examination before beginning any weight-reduction program that involves losing more than 15 to 20 pounds, taking regular medication, or adopting a very low-calorie diet (as is often the case with plans based on liquid formula that will replace your regular meals).

There is no reason why the doctor you consult for your medical exam cannot devise a weight-reduction and management plan for you. And it may be that you find a doctor who works with a dietitian or a nutritionist, so that you have some expert support and guidance over the coming months. However, it is equally likely that your doctor will not have the time, the expertise, or the personal interest to devote to the oversight of your weight-reduction program. Too often, you may find yourself given the generic advice to "watch what you eat and get more exercise." True enough, but it is precisely because following that advice is so excruciatingly difficult that the treatment of obesity has become a special discipline in its own right.

Sadly, many doctors are not doing everything they could and should do to flag the problems of obesity in patients who could benefit from weight-reduction counseling. A national survey of more than 12,000 obese adults by the Centers for Disease Control and Prevention found that less than half of them (42 percent) had been advised to lose weight during recent doctor visits for a routine checkup. Researchers found that the patients who were *most likely* to get this advice were middle-aged women who lived in the Northeast, were relatively more educated than the norm, and had diabetes and overall poorer health.[7] Thus it seems the ancient adage "The Lord helps those who help themselves" applies here. In the end, if you are battling obesity, you have more at stake than does your doctor. Be persistent and get the help you need.

> *In the end, if you are battling obesity, you have more at stake than does your doctor. Be persistent and get the help you need.*

WEIGHT-MANAGEMENT PROGRAMS AND CLINICS

If you want to take your quest to the next level, you would be well advised to look for a center or clinic that specializes in weight reduction.

At Johns Hopkins, a weight-management center was established in 1989. You will find such a center at a number of university hospitals, which are associated with medical schools, and at some regional and community hospitals. (See appendix.)

What to Expect

A comprehensive evaluation by a weight-management center should combine a number of different elements: a physical examination; a discussion of your medical history (which may be just as important and revelatory as the physical examination); tests by an exercise physiologist to determine your general level of fitness and how fast your body burns calories when you are sitting still (known as your *resting metabolic rate*); a meeting with a behavioral psychologist to discuss possible emotional or psychological factors involved in overeating; and a meeting with a dietitian or nutritionist to take an inventory of how much you are eating as well as what you are eating, and to devise a plan for improving your diet.

If nothing else, the fact that at least four different specialists will be involved in your assessment should underline the fact that obesity is not a simple problem. Nor is there one magic bullet that will stop obesity in its tracks.

The following are some of the questions you may be asked to answer as part of your consultation, or even in advance of your first appointment:

Medical history. Do you have any history of diabetes, thyroid disorder, high blood pressure, high cholesterol, cancer, heartburn, sleep difficulties, gallbladder disease, gout, ulcers (and more)? When and for what have you been hospitalized? Are you on any medications?

Family history. Are (or were) your parents, brothers, or sisters overweight? By how much? How about your spouse? Have any close relatives had any of the above diseases or disorders?

Eating habits. What foods do you crave most? Do you eat while watching TV? Do you eat breakfast? Do you eat before going to bed?

How often do you eat at fast-food restaurants, vending machines, cafeterias, hot dog or other quick-food stands, full-service restaurants? How often do you feel hungry? When do you feel most hungry? How many times a day do you eat meals? How many times a day do you snack?

Weight history. What was your weight, decade by decade, and by 5-year increments as a child? What's the most you ever weighed? When, and for how long? How often have you dieted? When? What kind of diet, and what were the results? For women: How much have you gained with pregnancies?

Health habits. Do you smoke (and how much)? Do you drink alcohol (and how much)? Do you use "recreational" drugs? Do you gamble? Do you ever shop in such a way that it becomes a problem? Do you participate in vigorous physical activities (such as running) or moderate physical activities (such as vacuuming or playing golf)?

Health-related quality-of-life assessment. How has your weight affected your health? Do you have physical limitations that are related to excess weight? Can you climb several flights of stairs? One flight of stairs? Can you walk several blocks? One block? Do you suffer from chronic pain?

These questions may sound intimidating, but they really should not be. You may well find that you begin making connections yourself for the first time as you scroll back through your life as a child and your subsequent medical history. You may be amazed when you start adding up all the times and places that you put food or drink into your mouth during the day. You may find the lightbulb going on when you think hard about when you are most hungry, and when and why you feel most like reaching for a candy bar or treating yourself with a bowl of ice cream. It's like putting together a jigsaw puzzle, where even the tiniest piece will be

> *You may well find that you begin making connections yourself for the first time as you scroll back through your life as a child and your subsequent medical history.*

needed for the picture to be complete. Everyone involved in the weight-management team—doctors, behavioral psychologists, exercise physiologists, dietitians and nutritionists—will need this information in order to devise the best possible individual plan for you. No two people are exactly alike.

A Comprehensive Assessment

A comprehensive assessment at the Johns Hopkins Weight Management Center typically includes all of the following tests and evaluations:

- A medical history, as just described, and a physical examination, with particular attention paid to those physical findings that may indicate a medical cause for weight gain (primarily, signs of a glandular or genetic disorder), or which are signs of conditions and diseases that occur more frequently in people who are obese (such as high blood pressure, osteoarthritis, or signs of heart or other diseases of the circulatory system). Often, blood tests are performed in conjunction with the medical examination, both as a screen for conditions which are not usually detectable during the medical examination (such as high cholesterol or other lipid problems), and to provide confirmation for or evidence against conditions which are suspected by the physician as a result of certain findings during the gathering of your medical history or in performing your physical exam (for example, if you report that you have noticed increasing thirst or urination, blood tests for diabetes will certainly be ordered by your doctor).

- A dietitian or nutritionist will focus on the specifics of your usual diet. This will include any issues with portion size, macronutrient content (that is, the proportion of your intake that is composed of fats versus proteins versus carbohydrates), and micronutrient adequacy (that is, whether your diet is sufficiently varied in order for you to obtain adequate amounts of essential vitamins and minerals), as well as patterns of eating such as snacking, skipping breakfast or other meals, and frequency of dining out and the use of "fast" foods. Instruments used may include food-frequency questionnaires (asking how often you eat various foods), assessment of food-preparation techniques and awareness, and 24-hour dietary recalls (what did you eat yesterday?) This part of the comprehensive assessment often is the time when measurements of weight, height, and waist circumference are made.

- Through a carefully structured interview, a behavioral psychologist or counselor will focus on the habits and other behavioral and psychological factors that influence your ability to control your body weight. These factors may include uncovering an eating disorder or depression. The existence of either of these conditions may sabotage your efforts at weight control and usually require special treatment or medications, which a physician can prescribe. Other areas typically delved into include assessing your readiness and motivators for seeking weight loss; the behaviors that trigger excessive eating when you are not physically hungry and which often derail weight-control efforts; and the existence of any barriers to weight control, including sabotage from family or friends.

> *A behavioral psychologist or counselor will focus on the habits and other behavioral and psychological factors that influence your ability to control your body weight.*

- An exercise physiologist or exercise counselor will focus on your current level of physical activity and fitness; often your fitness is assessed by measuring your pulse rate before and after you perform specific exercises. The exercise specialist is most accomplished in exploring what sorts of physical activities you might enjoy, as well as helping invigorate and sustain your interest in becoming more physically fit. At the Johns Hopkins Weight Management Center, the exercise physiologist uses a bioimpedance device to approximate your body-fat composition, and an indirect calorimetry machine to measure your metabolism (your resting metabolic rate). The calorimetry machine measures the amount of oxygen you consume and carbon dioxide you produce by sampling the air you exhale after an overnight fast, while you sit quietly under a clear plastic hood. Such testing can yield a much more precise, individualized indicator of the amount of calories you can consume in a day without gaining weight.

LINDA'S STORY: WHEN SCIENCE INTERVENES

Having been trained as a health professional did not prevent Linda Cartwright (not her real name) from becoming obese. More precisely, it did not prevent her from becoming even more obese than she already was—morbidly obese. Her education did not shield her from diabetes, loss of sight in one eye, sleep apnea, asthma, arthritis in both knees, and such an extreme degree of overweight that she was confined to her bedroom, all while still in her 40s.

Linda was always heavy, as far back as she could remember. Things had to get really ugly, however, before she turned to a comprehensive weight-control clinic, and started shedding enough pounds to regain some control over her life.

As she looks back, her lifelong struggle with weight began at birth, although she was only a 5-pound infant. "I had loose skin," she recounts, "and my grandmother said, 'Oh, she's going to be fat.'" If this was a prophecy, maybe it was of the self-fulfilling variety, because the other members of Linda's family took up the same mantra. "The family kept telling me, 'You're going to be fat, because you had loose skin.'" By the time she was in the fourth grade, Linda was "picking up weight and getting chubby—but not to the point where I wasn't functional."

But it was not long before Linda discovered what seemed like a positive reason to gain weight. She only realized the perversity of the logic many years later, after spending time with a psychologist specializing in obesity.

"Starting at the age of 12, my father used to come home drunk and start to fight with my mother," she says, with the 20-20 clarity of hindsight. "I could stand between my mother and my father, and hold my father off from getting to my mother with a hand on his chest—because I was taller than him, and I became bigger than him. My bigness made me able to hold my father away. So I believed in my soul, if I got big, I could handle things. This carried over into the rest of my life. When I graduated from the 12th grade, I was a size 18, which means I was already 185 to 200 pounds."

When Linda (who stands 5 feet, 8 inches) went to college, she ate while she studied. She ate while she wrote term papers. When she had a relationship with a man that ended badly, she ate to bury the hurt. All the while she was doing well in professional terms. She completed a bachelor's degree in biology and worked as a schoolteacher long enough to realize that was not the ideal profession for her. She studied medical technology and got a job in a blood bank, which she enjoyed until her fear of AIDS led her to look for another career.

She took another course of study and became a respiratory therapist. It was while she was working as a respiratory therapist, at age 29, that Linda gave birth to her only child, a son (now 19). Diabetes that she developed during the pregnancy led to retinal damage in her right eye, which now qualifies her as being legally blind.

By then, she tilted the scales at 350. She was still working hard to meet everybody's needs but her own, and she was still gaining weight, building that big buffer against the world.

> By the time she was in her late 30s, Linda was up to 468 pounds—at which point she literally collapsed, overcome with asthma, sleep apnea, and diabetes.

By the time she was in her late 30s, Linda had gained more than 100 additional pounds—at which point she literally collapsed, overcome with asthma, sleep apnea, and diabetes. "I'm a born-again

Christian," she says, "but the trauma at that time was so great, I could not implement my faith. I was overwhelmed, I was 468 pounds, and I collapsed. I gave up."

So it was in 1990, at the age of 37, that Linda went on disability. At first, she enjoyed kicking back and allowing others to look after her. She'd spent years, as the most educated member of her family, trying to take care of everyone else. Now the shoe was on the other foot.

But after a while, Linda's innate intelligence, education, and ambition got the best of her. She tried to "come out of the ditch that I'd created." Improbably, despite the strikes against her, she went back to school at a well-known urban university, took computer classes, and enrolled in a master's degree program in city and regional planning. She not only finished the degree, her research—on the plight of inner-city workers prevented from getting plum jobs in the suburbs because of the lack of mass transit—was interesting enough that it got picked up by a major national newspaper.

But jobs did not follow. "People don't want to hire obese people," she says today. "They consider them as health risks."

Perhaps inevitably, she responded as she always had—putting on more weight, thickening the buffer. And she physically withdrew from society. "What I did was retreat into my room, and I stayed in my room. I lived in my room."

Ironically, when she was a respiratory therapist, she had a patient who resembled the person she became. "I met a lady who was so obese she could not walk," Linda recalls, "and I had to give her treatments. I had a fear that I would get as big as her one day. To me, she was kind of helpless. She depended on everybody to do everything for her, because she could not get out of bed, and I had a fear of that. But over the years, when I accepted disability as a lifestyle, I became comfortable with that and I was creating the same situation that I had feared.

"I didn't leave my bed, except to go to the bathroom. I had the TV, I had the remote control, I had the computer, I had everything within reach. I would call my family—call my niece or call my son—

to bring me water, bring me food, do this for me, do that for me, and they would cater to me. When I went to family gatherings, all I had to do was walk in the house and sit down, and they would fix my food and bring it to me. I had created a world where I didn't have to do anything, because I had everybody enabling me to stay disabled."

And still, the weight crept up—from 468 to 480, to 500, to 519—her personal peak. "So here I am now in my 40s, at 519 and having trouble walking."

Increasingly, Linda's life became intolerable to her. But when she read the book *Who Moved My Cheese?*, a bestselling fable about how so many people are resistant to change, she decided something had to give. "I came out of whatever I was in, and said, 'I don't want to live like this. There is no reason why I cannot have a house, a job, a car, and live a life other than in these four walls.' I started praying."

Her first step, literally and metaphorically, was deciding she had to spend part of each day outside of her bedroom. "I moved stuff out of my room and made my room a bedroom. So I get up in the morning and make up my bed and I live in other parts of my house, and I don't get back into bed until I am ready to go to sleep. That one decision let me dare to press on to do other things in my life."

First and foremost was to go talk to her personal doctor. "I said, 'Look, I can't walk. I have pains shooting up and down my legs and my back hurts. It's so easy for me to lie in bed because it's too painful to even get up and stand and walk. I get short of breath going from my bedroom to the bathroom to the kitchen. You need to help me.'"

But Linda's doctor told her that her Medicare coverage would not pay for weight-loss treatment (although Medicare *would* pay for a $10,000 gastric bypass operation that Linda wanted to avoid (see

> *I didn't leave my bed, except to go to the bathroom. I had the TV, I had the remote control, I had the computer, I had everything within reach. I would call my family—call my niece or call my son—to bring me water, bring me food, do this for me, do that for me, and they would cater to me.*
>
> —LINDA

chapter 5, "Surgery," for more on that procedure). Linda's doctor said her options were to stop eating so much or to talk to a nutritionist. After a fruitless trip to a psychiatrist—for which Medicare paid 50 percent of the bill—Linda cut a deal with her state's Department of Rehabilitation. She convinced her disability caseworker to pay for a comprehensive assessment of her condition at a university weight-management clinic—a program Linda had found in her own hometown through hours of research on the Internet.

"It deals with the medical, the diet, the exercise, the psychological, even the spiritual—if you want to put it that way," says Linda. "You have a program that deals with the whole person, to bring them to the point of life transformation."

> *Within 4 months of entering the program, Linda had lost 50 pounds and she was still losing weight. Her weight loss was based on both physiological and psychological insights, as well as a strict, medically supervised diet plan.*

Within 4 months of entering the program, Linda had lost 50 pounds and she was still losing weight. Her weight loss was based on both physiological and psychological insights, as well as a strict, medically supervised diet plan.

An exercise physiologist tested her respiration to determine the rate at which she burns calories sitting still. Linda learned that she has a relatively low rate of metabolism. She needs a little over 2,000 calories per day at rest to maintain her weight at 500 pounds. Along with the dietitian and the physician, the exercise physiologist recommended that she go on an 1,100-calorie-per-day diet, which will enable her to lose weight steadily.

The exercise physiologist also showed Linda some videotapes that illustrated calorie-burning exercises she can do while sitting in her chair or swimming in a pool, which Linda enjoys because water helps to support her weight.

The dietitian helped Linda take systematic stock of everything she ate, every day. For the first time in her life, Linda kept a written record of all the calories that went in her mouth, in whatever form.

Under the medically supervised diet, she is allowed to take five specially designed dietary supplements a day and to cook one ordinary meal for herself, consisting of four ounces of meat and vegetables chosen from an approved list. The supplements come in shake, nutrition bar, soup, and hot chocolate form, and Linda finds them tasty. "The diet is good because you're never hungry," she says. "It makes you feel full."

The psychologist helped Linda achieve the insight discussed earlier—that she had gained weight as a way of trying to deal with challenges in her life by "getting bigger." The follow-up weekly group-therapy meetings have helped Linda realize that she is not alone—she empathizes with her fellow dieter who cannot pass a fast-food restaurant at night without pulling in for a snack of chicken wings, even though she knows they're bad for her. And having to report in every week makes Linda stick to her diet. "If you have to go in and weigh yourself and give a list of what you ate all week, it makes you accountable. You say, 'I can't be cheating, because I've got to face these people.'"

Linda knows she is not out of the woods, but for the first time in many years, she has acquired a sense of insight and confidence. "I told the doctor that I don't want to be on a diet just as a way to lose weight," she says. "I am looking at it as a lifestyle—that once I achieve my weight loss, I can keep making wise choices in my life, keep the weight off, and stay healthy. That's my decision."

And for the first time in many years, she is able to do something as ordinary as shop in the grocery store, come home, and cook a meal—

> *Linda knows she is not out of the woods, but for the first time in many years, she has acquired a sense of insight and confidence.*

without requiring, literally, two days of recovery from the outing. "I'm still sitting up, I'm still active, my feet are not swollen, and I feel great," she said. "Losing 50 pounds has helped me a lot. It makes a real difference. It's an accomplishment."

SUMMARY

If you've done the tape-measure test and found your waist exceeds the cutoffs described earlier, or if you discovered that your BMI is 30 or above—well, join the club. Unfortunately, it's a large one. Over half of American adults are overweight or obese. Maybe you will have the discipline to cut out all those midmorning danishes, afternoon candy bars, and postdinner bowls of ice cream. Maybe seeing the unpleasant numbers will steel your will to leave the house for a brisk half-hour walk or jog, each and every day. But if not, help is available. The best place to start is with a comprehensive medical evaluation. What comes next will depend on your success in dieting under a doctor's tutelage, risk factors, and degree of obesity, among other considerations. For a discussion of treatment options, read on.

CHAPTER 3

Diet and Exercise
Can You Lose Weight Without Them?

⁂

AT ANY GIVEN time, surveys say, about 25 percent of American men and 40 percent of American women are trying to lose weight. In practice, this usually means that we are trying to follow a diet of some kind. At an intuitive level, we understand that if we want to shed pounds and inches, we need to eat less food. Whether we also understand that we need to increase our physical-activity level to include at least 30 minutes of vigorous exercise per day is another question. But unless we do both together, it is very unlikely that we can sustain our weight-loss goals over time—even if we can drop an initial 10 or 20 pounds through sheer willpower and self-denial.

Although there have been literally hundreds, if not thousands, of named diet plans that have gained some measure of popular favor, it is important to know that we are now in the position of understanding more about diets and *why they fail* than ever before. We know less, perhaps, about why some people are able to succeed more quickly or more easily than others, though it is clear that genetic differences in people's metabolisms and fat-storing efficiency help to explain why the same diet can work so well for one person and fail for another. Also bear in mind the fact that a small percentage of obese people are overweight because of medical conditions that they cannot control, as discussed earlier. That is why you should begin with a thorough physical evaluation by a doctor if you want to lose a substantial amount of weight.

Nevertheless, consider the basic reality of the relationship between calories and weight. If we take in more energy than we expend, that excess energy will be stored in our bodies as fat. Genetic differences between people do not alter that fundamental maxim, although they may account for varying degrees of *efficiency* in accomplishing the storage.

Among the things that we understand better now are the following:

- Why pounds can be shed so quickly in the early weeks of a diet
- Why weight loss then so often comes to a frustrating halt, or "plateau"
- How to break through the plateau and resume weight loss
- The importance of professional counseling and peer-to-peer support groups for establishing new behavior patterns in relation to food and exercise
- How to set realistic goals for weight reduction that will allow you to be successful and improve your health—as opposed to "crashing and burning" in the pursuit of unrealistic Hollywood ideals

Researchers also have achieved fascinating insights into the everyday, winning strategies of people who have been able to lose large amounts of weight and keep it off without either drugs or surgery.

Most of this perspective is based on work that began about half a century ago, in the early 1950s, when the medical community began to explore aggressive treatments for those suffering from obesity.

These early medical attempts to treat obese patients embraced an initial trial of total fasting (starvation) as an appropriate means of reducing body fat. But doctors soon found that while they were able to induce aggressive weight loss (for a short period of time), there were many adverse effects on health and, occasionally, death resulted. Enthusiasm for this type of regime gradually waned. On the one hand, it was difficult to maintain a starvation diet on an outpatient basis, for obvious reasons; on the other hand, however, inpatient therapy—with the patient checked into a hospital or clinic for the course of treatment—was too expensive for widespread use. However, the idea of the severely restricted diet as a cure for the obese continued to captivate the medical community. As research continued, and the understanding of human nutrition and metabolism increased, diets became more calculated and were often prescribed to provide specific calorie levels as well as measured amounts of protein and carbohydrate.

> *Researchers also have achieved fascinating insights into the everyday, winning strategies of people who have been able to lose large amounts of weight and keep it off without either drugs or surgery.*

Researchers noted that the same rapid loss of weight could occur with the addition of small amounts of nutrients. So the idea of modified fasting was born, which led to the development of the Very Low Calorie Diet (VLCD), also referred to as the Very Low Energy Diet (VLED).

VERY LOW CALORIE DIETS

Today, the use of structured Very Low Calorie Diet (VLCD) plans by the medical community is administered in both inpatient and outpatient settings, but are usually hospital-based and require frequent contact with medical practitioners.

This is one aspect of weight control where the following warning is warranted: *Don't try this at home.* Medical supervision is definitely required. Many eating disorders are, in a sense, self-administered VLCDs, all too often with disastrous results.

Side Effects of VLCDs

Severe restriction of a person's caloric intake (which is to say, clamping down on the consumption of all food and drink other than water) creates predictable changes in the body's metabolism, including the following:

- A slower metabolic rate. Paradoxically, at just the time we most want our body to burn fat and shed pounds, it reacts to the rapid decline in food intake by *decreasing* the rate at which it burns fat! This is actually a defensive mechanism designed to protect us against starvation by conserving our energy stores, and it is a key reason why rapid, sustained weight loss is so difficult.
- Increased loss of lean body mass, such as muscle tissue.
- Loss of electrolytes such as sodium and potassium, leading to fatigue, low blood pressure, muscle cramps and weakness, anorexia, diarrhea, heart irregularities, vomiting, and mental clouding.
- Elevated uric acid, which may precipitate the development of kidney stones.
- Anemia
- The development of stones in the gallbladder.

People consuming VLCDs may also experience headache, fruity breath, dizziness, nausea, and cold intolerance. As with most low-calorie diets, dry skin and hair loss are possible consequences. Most of these symptoms will diminish when calories are increased.

> *Many eating disorders are, in a sense, self-administered VLCDs, all too often with disastrous results.*

There are, however, some positive side effects of VLCDs. These positive side effects occur due to a change in the way the body utilizes energy. Under normal conditions, the body will use a combination of all three major nutrients in foods (carbohydrate, fat, and protein) as fuels. However, when nutrient intake is changed by dieting (that is, when calories and carbohydrates are restricted), the body will adapt and begin to burn the fuels available (adipose or fat tissue). As fat becomes the major source for energy, there is an increased production of ketones (a byproduct of fat's chemical breakdown, or catabolism, within the body). After approximately 3 days of increased fat catabolism, there is a sufficient amount of ketones in the blood to curb hunger and create a mild sense of improved well-being, which patients often refer to as having increased "energy." These particular side effects may play a role in maintaining adherence to the VLCD.

How Low It Can Go: Defining the VLCD

Total energy intake is often restricted to less than 800 calories per day, with minimum amounts of calories varying from 330 to 400 for women[1] and 500 for men.[2] Other attempts at defining the most effective VLCDs have led to an individual approach where calorie needs are determined based upon the ideal body weight (IBW) of the patient.

The structure of the VLCD has also evolved from simply providing calories, irrespective of their food group, to providing calories with specific amounts of protein. There is also a consensus that protein of high biological value providing all of the essential amino acids (in general, animal sources instead of plant sources) is critical to helping preserve lean body mass such as muscle tissue and organs. Recommendations concerning the amount of daily protein vary widely, from a minimum of 40 grams to the very high levels of 1.2 to 1.5 grams per kilogram of IBW. Optimal amounts of carbohydrate are also unknown and ranges vary from small (20 grams per day) to moderate (100 grams per day) amounts. If the diet provided uses whole foods, the consumption of very lean meats, egg whites, and other lowfat sources of protein with small amounts of low-calorie vegetables is required. Because of the decreased variety and need for the severe restriction or total omission of several basic food groups (dairy, fruit, and grain products), it is often necessary to provide vitamin, mineral, and fiber supplements. Meal replacements, such as specially formulated milk shakes, fruit drinks, and food bars may also be used to improve the nutrient intake of the patient and increase the variety of the diet. The use of fortified meal-replacement products can also help to ensure that the minimum daily nutrient needs (100 percent of the recommended daily allowances, or RDAs) are met while aggressive weight loss is pursued.

How Well Does the VLCD Work?

The rate of weight loss will depend upon the size of the individual and the degree of calorie deficit induced by the particular weight-loss plan. For example, on a VLCD of 800 calories per day, a 350-pound man who typically burns 2,800 calories per day will have a calorie deficit of 2,000 calories per day. In theory, there are 3,500 calories in each pound of human fat; therefore, this dieter could expect an approximate loss of 4 pounds of adipose tissue (fat) per week. The same diet administered to a 200-pound woman who typically burns 2,100 calories a day would induce a loss of approximately 2.6 pounds of adipose tissue per week. The magnitude or total amount of weight loss is dependent upon many factors that will vary from person to person, such as compliance (how rigorously one observes the caloric limits called for in the diet), exercise, and duration of the program.

> A recent review of 29 studies of overweight and obese people who participated in weight-loss programs in the United States found that supplement-based VLCDs are effective for both weight loss and maintenance.

A recent review of 29 studies of overweight and obese people who participated in weight-loss programs in the United States found that supplement-based VLCDs are effective for both weight loss and maintenance.[3] Adults who followed a VLCD were able to lose significantly more weight and maintained the loss for a greater length of time (over 5 years) than comparable subjects following a more traditional food-based plan of 1,200 to 1,500 calories per day. The study noted that after one year, those on a VLCD (utilizing shakes, energy bars, and low-calorie entrees) decreased their weight by 16 percent compared to those who followed a low-energy food-based plan, who averaged a 7 percent loss. Follow-up after 5 years showed that the VLCD dieters had also maintained a greater loss of 6 percent, compared with 2 percent for the food dieters. So it appears that supplement-based diets are at least as effective and certainly as appropriate as other dieting measures.

Who Should Use VLCDs?

Although VLCDs have been proven effective for short periods of time, they are usually not embraced by the medical community as standard practice. Many doctors now believe that severe calorie restriction is not any more effective than the slightly increased calorie intake seen with Low Calorie Diets (LCDs) and are less willing to prescribe and administer VLCD programs. Given this view, it is important that patients be carefully selected based on their degree of obesity (usually a BMI of 30 or above), as well as their medical history (such as whether there is the presence of heart disease, diabetes, and hypertension). The presence of these types of medical conditions may add to the argument for the more aggressive weight-loss program, as they usually lessen in severity or disappear altogether as weight is lost. Contraindications such as a recent heart attack, liver and kidney disease, diabetes that is not well controlled, and pregnancy must also be evaluated as well as psychological conditions such as binge eating, purging, and manic-depressive disorder. Side effects (including electrolyte changes, dehydration, and constipation) must be treated. Careful monitoring is necessary and physician involvement is recommended to adjust medications and attend to side effects as they develop. Follow-up interventions vary and often parallel those of more conventional weight-loss plans.

LOW CALORIE DIETS

Low Calorie Diets (LCDs) are defined as those providing greater than 800 calories per day. As with the VLCD, the actual amount of calories that determines an LCD is individual and based upon the metabolic expenditure (or calories burned) on a daily basis. For the sake of discussion, and as is consistent with usual practice, the LCD is usually defined as allowing between 800 and 1,200 calories per day. In order to decrease the loss of lean body mass, the amount of protein provided in the diet is usually high. Fat content is low, as well as the carbohydrate level, which can be low enough to induce a state of ketosis (less than 100 grams per day), as seen with the VLCD. The majority of diet plans are supplement-based and comprised of a variety of shakes, food bars, soups and, occasionally, cereals and pasta dishes. Though controversy exists within the medical community about the efficacy of this type of diet (also referred to as a protein-sparing, modified fast), it is employed by numerous obesity-treatment centers and has been shown to be effective to achieve weight loss for the management as well as prevention of medical complications such as diabetes, hypertension, and heart disease.

Recent studies have confirmed that these types of programs are effective and that weight loss can be sustained. After weight loss is achieved and food is reintroduced and supplement use is decreased, it is important for patients to understand that their program is not over. Success will depend upon their ability to sustain their loss. In order to do this, they will need to develop a maintenance plan and to address nutrition and behavioral issues that have been placed on the back burner during the supplement phase of the plan. Though there is a definite place for LCDs in the arsenal of weight-loss techniques, meal-replacement programs do little to help obese people learn to cope with food and the behaviors that go with eating in ordinary, day-to-day settings. When a significant weight loss has been dependent upon meal-replacement products and supplements, it may not have been founded on new dietary patterns or on an increased un-

> *Though there is a definite place for LCDs in the arsenal of weight-loss techniques, meal-replacement programs do little to help obese people learn to cope with food and the behaviors that go with eating in ordinary, day-to-day settings.*

derstanding of foods, fats, and calories. Nor will people on these types of programs be able to identify their own individual triggers for overeating and then develop alternative behaviors. Without these skills in place, people will return to previous behaviors surrounding their food habits and ultimately regain their lost weight.

Side Effects of Low Calorie Diets

The side effects of LCDs, as is the case with any severe restriction of food intake, may vary from poor vitamin and mineral intake leading to various forms of malnutrition, to those side effects seen with the VLCD, including fatigue, headache, constipation, dry skin, and hair loss. Due to the risk of changes in blood pressure, the development of gallstones, and the need to adjust medications as weight is lost, those undertaking the LCD should be medically supervised. Side effects should be monitored and treated to maintain optimal health and well-being.

What the Low Calorie Diet Looks Like

The LCD, like the VLCD, is designed to be an aggressive treatment for weight loss. If whole foods are to be used, as opposed to specially formulated meal replacements, the diet will resemble the VLCD, with larger portions. Foods are usually restricted to lean proteins and vegetables, the goal being to eat the most amount of food while ingesting the least amount of calories. Because of the monotony of the diet as well as nutrient insufficiencies, LCDs are most often provided in the form of meal replacements fortified with vitamins, minerals, and fiber as well as electrolytes such as sodium and potassium. Many commercial food-supplement programs are available. Daily eating is centered around four to five meal replacements such as shakes, fruit-flavored drinks, food bars, and soups, which are taken approximately every 3 to 4 hours. A small meal may also be included, consisting of lean protein and salad or vegetable. In order to lessen the incidence of gallstones, a tablespoon of fat or oil (100 calories) is also recommended in the meal plan.

When Should LCDs Be Used?

LCDs are for the benefit of those who have a BMI greater than 30, or a lower BMI accompanied by debilitating medical conditions that would improve significantly with weight loss. LCDs are also warranted when a more aggressive weight loss is desired, as in preparation for surgery. The selection of appropriate patients for the LCD plan is complex. Other considerations include use of and success on previous LCD plans, commitment to the re-feeding phase after weight loss has been achieved, presence or absence of major life stresses, a history of eating disorders as well as the presence of severe depression or other mental illness. It is highly recommended that LCDs be medically supervised and that they be provided as a part of a multidisciplinary program that addresses behavioral as well as exercise therapies to achieve long-term success.

> *LCDs are for the benefit of those who have a BMI greater than 30, or a lower BMI accompanied by debilitating medical conditions that would improve significantly with weight loss.*

How Well Does the LCD Work?

LCDs are well known to be capable of producing large weight losses of 2 to 5 pounds or more per week during the first 2 weeks, mostly due to the loss of fluid from body tissues. During this early dieting phase, the body is using up its stores of carbohydrate (glycogen) and, as it does, water is released and lost in the urine. This is, generally speaking, the basis of any strict diet's relatively rapid weight loss in the first couple of weeks. As the body enters the state of ketosis, "weight loss" slows and will decrease to a rate dependent upon the calories-in and calories-out equation. With strict adherence to the caloric limit and increased burning of calories with exercise, weight loss can be sustained at an increased rate. The actual amount lost each week is dependent upon the size of the individual. Those with greater fat mass as well as greater lean body mass will lose at a faster rate. For example, people with 100 to 200 pounds of adipose tissue will lose more quickly than those with only 50 pounds of adipose tissue, as will those with greater muscle mass, such as males.

As with any weight-loss diet, the rate of loss is variable depending upon the individual's metabolic rate, the size of the caloric deficit induced by the LCD, the amount of adipose tissue at the start of the plan, and the amount of calories burned in resting metabolism as well as through exercise. Most people can expect to lose an average of 2 to 4 pounds per week after the initial loss in water weight. Recent studies have strengthened the argument that supplement-based low-calorie diets are effective for weight loss and that lower weight can be maintained for an extended period of time (see comments in VLCD section).

DEFINING SUCCESS

Success in the world of weight management is a difficult concept to define. Increasingly, it is obvious that weight-loss professionals have a different definition of success than do most people who are trying to lose weight. It is not unusual for obese women, for instance, to want to regain the size 6 they wore when they left high school, or on the day they got married. Twenty years on, that ambition may not be realistic for many people. Failure to achieve an unrealistic goal after some period of dieting may lead to discouragement, depression, and a relapse to old eating habits, followed by weight regain. But most doctors have a different understanding of what is realistically achievable, and they prefer to set weight-loss goals that would be beneficial in terms of health. Current research suggests that a loss of 5 to 10 percent of initial body weight is successful, in that it appears to afford most overweight people profound health benefits.[4] Thus, for instance, if a 300-pound man can permanently lose 15 to 30 pounds, he will be significantly better off from a health standpoint. The same holds true for a 200-pound woman losing 10 to 20 pounds—and keeping it off.

As may be becoming clear, a crucial indicator of success for any weight-loss plan is the length of time for which the weight loss is maintained. It is not uncommon to hear people say that they reached their goal weight on a weight-loss plans for "one minute" and then began the upward climb to their previous level of obesity. Is this success? It appears that the previous diet worked for as long as it was followed. However, the diet was dropped like a hot potato the moment the dieter crossed the goal line. But the game (to extend the metaphor) was only in the first quarter—way too early to stop playing.

> *Increasingly, it is obvious that weight-loss professionals have a different definition of success than do most people who are trying to lose weight.*

More realistically, success should be defined as reaching and *maintaining* a lower body weight, even if that the loss is only 10 pounds. Success will depend upon ongoing support. As health-care professionals help the patient to focus on the importance of the "post-diet" phase of a weight-management program and provide support and help in improving skills, success will be maintained for longer periods of time.

PLATEAUING

The single most important motivator for anyone following a diet program is measuring the amount of weight loss. Some people can't wait to climb on the scales daily to chart their progress; others, weekly.

All dieters look forward to seeing the results of their hard work, and all dieters focus on the number on the scale as a sign of their success. Then, for no apparent reason, the scale refuses to budge. Feelings of disappointment rise. This event, which can occur at any time during any weight-loss program, has been coined a "weight-loss plateau."

So, what can be done to overcome the plateau and get on with weight loss? One of the biggest causes of weight-loss plateaus is that

> **How and When to Weigh Yourself**
>
> Monitoring your progress is an important aspect of any weight-loss and weight-maintenance program. It is recommended that you weigh yourself once a week. It makes no difference where you weigh yourself unless you weigh naked or require a scale that will hold in excess of 350 pounds (most scales for home use are limited in the number of pounds they will weigh). Digital scales are easier to read and many have a monitor that is extended up from the standing platform where there is less struggle to view the numbers. When you weigh yourself probably doesn't matter, but it may be important to weigh at the same time each week (such as Saturday at 9 A.M.). Weight can fluctuate throughout the day and may vary depending upon the fullness of your bladder and how much food and fluid you have recently consumed. For example, a liter of fluid weighs 2.2 pounds. If you drink the fluid right before you weigh yourself, you will be 2.2 pounds heavier. Weighing on a daily basis may be discouraging, as day-to-day changes may be small. Most clinicians recommend weighing on a weekly basis, as the progress displayed on the scales may be more rewarding.

dieters stop paying enough attention to what and how much they are eating.

Some solutions to a weight-loss plateau follow.

Write down everything you are eating. This is known as maintaining a food record or food log. A food record or food log is usually a type of journal or diary for tracking foods that are eaten daily or on specific days. It is a very important tool for success and can give you insightful information about what, when, where, how much, and sometimes why you eat. In addition to increasing awareness, the food log can be a source of external accountability (causing you to think twice before eating a particular food, knowing that you will need to record it in your diary). It may be easier to carry a small pocket pad and then transfer to a diary (to examine fat and calorie content) later in the day. However you choose to maintain your diary, it is important to remember to:

> One of the biggest causes of weight-loss plateaus is that dieters stop paying enough attention to what and how much they are eating.

1. Write down everything you eat and drink, even small bites.
2. Note how a food was prepared (such as "breaded and fried") and record details, including condiments (mayonnaise vs. mustard) and whether a beverage was sweetened or unsweetened.
3. Record foods as they are eaten whenever possible.
4. Be sure to complete your diary by filling in fat grams and calories.
5. Consider using the diary to note hunger and fullness as well as other emotions surrounding your meals and snacks.

Measure your foods. Make sure the portions are within your recommended size and calorie limits. Any type of measuring cups or spoons will work for measuring foods at home. A simple food scale for weighing may also be helpful. Recommended portion sizes can be the amount listed as a portion on a label; the amount providing a certain amount of calories; the amount deemed appropriate according to the Food Guide Pyramid; or the amount recommended by a weight-loss counselor. The American Dietetic Association offers the following familiar comparisons:

- Three ounces of meat, poultry, or fish is about the size of a deck of playing cards, or the size of the palm of a woman's hand, or the size of a computer mouse.
- A half-cup of pasta, rice, or mashed potatoes, or cut fruit or vegetables, is about the size of a small fist.

- One cup of yogurt or chopped fresh greens is about the size of a small hand holding a tennis ball.
- One ounce of cheese is the size of your thumb.
- An average bagel is the size of a hockey puck.
- An ounce of snack foods (pretzels, etc.) equals a large handful.[5]

Check the calorie content of the foods you are choosing. Use food labels, calorie and fat guides (many are pocket-size for convenience and availability)—as well as the Internet—to increase your knowledge and understanding of both appropriate portion sizes and calorie content. Software programs are now available for handheld computers, such as Palm Pilots, that not only provide a guide to the calorie content of foods but also allow you to enter the foods into a log and calculate your daily intake. It may also be helpful to look at recipes and see if there are high-calorie ingredients involved in preparation. If dining out, consider checking out the foods before you dine. For example, if you plan to eat Asian, look up the calorie and fat content of several dishes and go prepared to make better choices. And don't forget to check the calories in beverages (wine, mixed drinks, and so on).

Many dieters will be surprised to find that they have gradually increased the amount of food they are consuming. And some will find that they are snacking a little more than they realized. Any or all of the preceding evaluation techniques may help to uncover the cause of a plateau. Without a doubt, they are worth the added effort to get back on the road to weight loss.

At the opposite end of possible reasons for plateauing—and this will sound totally paradoxical—is that you are not eating enough calories. As we mentioned previously, overrestriction of energy intake can put our bodies into a starvation mode, which will further lower our metabolic rate and thwart our attempt at loss. The following are some solutions for this particular problem.

> *At the opposite end of possible reasons for plateauing—and this will sound totally paradoxical—is that you are not eating enough calories.*

Commit to eating at least 1,200 calories each day. Consider having your metabolic rate checked at a medically based weight-management center, using a metabolic cart. This is a test that measures the amount of oxygen you use to determine the number of calories your body burns on a daily basis. You might be surprised to learn that your body may actually need more calories than you are consuming in order to meet its daily demands, and this information can be useful in ensuring you are taking in enough food to fuel your exercise and activity.

Check your exercise regime. As time goes by, many of us become lax with our exercise plan just as we can with our food plan. Maybe entire days are starting to slide by without the daily walk we started to take. Or maybe we are back to punching the button for the elevator instead of heading to the stairs. Maintain an activity and exercise log similar to or in addition to your food log. Recording your daily activities allows you to reevaluate your efforts and make the necessary changes to resume weight loss.

Increase your lean body mass by building more muscle. An excessive loss of muscle mass is another possible explanation for a stalled weight-loss program. When muscle mass (our calorie burner) is lost, you will need to consume even fewer calories in order to lose weight than when you first began your program. Add resistance or weight training to your exercise regime or consider increasing the intensity of your current program.

SET POINT THEORY

Throughout history it has been observed that people in any society become obese as soon as enough food and leisure time are available, leading to the conclusion that increased calorie intake or decreased energy expenditure lead to increased adiposity. Although this statement is true for a large segment of the population, we know that the development of severe obesity is not quite so simple. The reasons are complex and often related to genetic and psychological factors as well as being reflective of the socioeconomic and cultural environment. During the past 30 to 40 years, researchers' interest in determining the causes of severe obesity has increased as they seek to shed light on the development of effective treatments. Though a change in energy balance achieved by eating less and exercising more is an effective therapy for many, it has proven to be all but impossible for some. We have come to realize that not everyone will be able to achieve an "ideal body weight."

Interestingly, close observation of the eating habits of severely obese people has not confirmed that, as a group, they consume excessive amounts of calories, nor do they have a preference for higher-calorie foods when compared to normal-weight people. Speculation as to what creates severe obesity (as some people clearly are more susceptible than others) has led to the development of various theories, most of which now center on the increased understanding of our genetic makeup. The knowledge gained from these studies have led to the labeling of obesity as a medical condition, which causes us to view it more as a treatable entity requiring medical intervention and not merely an expression of gluttony and laziness gone awry.

One of the earlier and more pervasive theories is the notion of a "set point," which assumes that there is an active regulatory system within each of us that determines our body weight and that if left to our own devices, our body will attain and maintain that particular weight. This view of weight regulation was based on the observation that when you gain weight, your metabolism increases so you burn more calories, and when you lose weight, your metabolism decreases so you burn fewer calories. Your body makes the attempt to maintain a specific weight, or a "set point." Some of us have set points (predetermined body masses or resting metabolic rates) that lead to greater adiposity, and some of us appear to have set points that promote

> *Interestingly, close observation of the eating habits of severely obese people have not confirmed that, as a group, they consume excessive amounts of calories, nor do they have a preference for higher-calorie foods when compared to normal-weight people.*

a lower body mass. Speculation concerning the mechanisms regulating the "set point" include neurotransmitters in the brain, peptides in the liver and gut, proteins secreted by adipose tissue, and endocrine hormones such as insulin. These mechanisms, though powerful, are not immune to environmental factors. Certainly the great diversity of human body weight and the significant weight changes seen in many people during their lifetime would lead us to believe that these internally dictated numbers can change for each of us. In other words, it would appear that, if there is a "set point," it can be "reset" during the course of our lives.

Not only can body weight change in accordance with life events, it can change while a fetus is still in the womb. During the Dutch famine of World War II, the effects of a low-energy intake on the developing fetus were expressed in the subsequent prevalence of obesity during childhood, adolescence, and adulthood. The Dutch famine study was a type of natural "experiment" that occurred near the end of World War II as retribution for subversive activities against the Germans.[6] Food was restricted for most of the population of northern Holland for approximately 6 months, from about 1,500 calories per day to about 1,000 calories per day and then to about 500 calories per day. Dutch women who experienced famine in their last trimester (thought to be significant in that the last trimester is when fat cells are replicating and the fetus has a rapid increase in body fat) produced children who had a *reduced* incidence of obesity at 18 years. Women who were exposed to famine in the first two trimesters produced children with an *increased* prevalence of obesity. It was thought that the famine caused improper development of the hypothalamus, which regulates the response to caloric intake. The study is not perfect but certainly suggests that there are factors operating during gestation that may affect subsequent adiposity.

Obviously, whether any one person becomes obese is multifactorial, and this area of research concerning cause remains controversial. There is no doubt that more studies are needed before scientists can say with certainty that a person's genes may set limits on how much weight can be lost and maintained. And in spite of the great variation in relationships between caloric intake, energy expenditure, and body mass, it remains clear that there is a direct relationship between the increased availability of food, more leisure time spent in sedentary activities such as television viewing, and the problem of obesity.

And though the simple equation:

calories in < calories out = weight loss

does not predict the end results of dieting for any one specific individual, it remains the basic tenet of almost all weight-loss programs.

Because of the growing concern over the epidemic of overweight people in our society, new and diverse theories of obesity are being developed and explored. Of interest is a recent presentation at the 2001 American Chemical Society meeting by Sarah Leibowitz, an associate professor of neurobiology at The Rockefeller University in New York City. Her research in animal models (rats) suggests that eating a high-fat diet (as many Americans do) may trigger the brain to produce neurochemicals that can alter eating behaviors and body weight. When eaten, dietary fats, known as triglycerides, may stimulate the production of a cascade of chemicals, which may in turn interfere with the feeling of fullness (leading to overeating) and enhance fat storage. Leibowitz noted that a single high-fat meal was sufficient to stimulate the "fat-responsive" genes that produce overeating.[7]

> *Obviously, whether any one person becomes obese is multifactorial, and this area of research concerning cause remains controversial. There is no doubt that more studies are needed before scientists can say with certainty that a person's genes may set limits on how much weight can be lost and maintained.*

OTHER SUCCESSFUL METHODS OF REDUCING WEIGHT

Any plan that promotes gradual changes toward healthier eating habits will result in success. The key is to have a plan. Of those long-term successful dieters in the National Weight Loss Registry (which is explained later in this chapter), half are not members of any type of structured weight-management program, whereas the other half are. Some utilize popular programs such as Weight Watchers and Overeaters Anonymous; others became involved in various weight-loss clinics or sought individual counseling sessions with psychologists or dietitians. Approximately one-fifth of the participants in the registry used liquid-formula programs. Significantly, very few used fad diets (including the popular "high protein, low carbohydrate" plans) or weight-loss medications.

How to Spot a Fad Diet from a Mile Away

The word *fad* implies something of temporary importance, to be embraced passionately for only a short period of time. And so we have a vivid picture of "fad dieting." We all know what fad diets are and most likely we have followed one—probably for a short period of time! What we have come to know in the last 40 to 50 years in dieting history is that fad diets can be ineffective at their best and dangerous to our health at their worst. Multiple reliable health organizations, including the American Dietetic Association, the American Heart Association, and the USDA, have published scientifically based recommendations for safe and effective weight loss. Credible nutrition information is available everywhere (although rarely on the cover of the latest magazines you pass in the supermarket checkout line).

Before embarking upon any weight-loss program, apply the following guidelines to help determine whether the program is safe and will provide accurate and appropriate information to assist you in reaching your goals:

- Does the diet violate the principles of good nutrition? Is it designed to provide a wide variety of foods to ensure nutritional adequacy?

The majority of professional weight-loss counselors promote a threefold approach to success: behavioral changes, food and diet changes, and exercise. Skill building is important and includes the following:

1. Keeping a record of foods and beverages eaten each day.
2. Having an awareness of the caloric content or the appropriate portion size of foods.
3. Knowing how to evaluate foods for their fat and calorie content.

- Is there a claim for quick results and rapid weight loss (greater than 2 pounds per week)?
- Are there dramatic claims based on unsupported scientific research (recommendations based on a single study, refuted by reputable scientific organizations, or published without peer review)?
- Does the diet plan imply that weight can be lost and maintained without exercise and behavioral changes?
- Is there a warning for people with either diabetes or high blood pressure to seek advice from their health-care provider?

Diet plans can work. But it pays to be skeptical and to realize that the ultimate goals for achievement in any weight-loss program remain the following:

- Improved health and well-being
- Lifelong changes in the types and amounts of foods you eat
- Lifetime commitment to activity and exercise
- Permanent changes in food-related behaviors

These skills will help you to understand how many calories you may be eating on a regular basis, as well as helping you track the amount of fat consumed. They may also aid you in evaluating your diet for adequate amounts of calcium (dairy servings), protein (meat group), and phytochemicals (fruit and vegetable servings), as well as highlight areas of inappropriate eating.

Planning is also an essential skill to ensure success and includes the following:

1. Providing and preparing appropriate meals.

2. Keeping appropriate snacks available.

3. Being prepared for social events.

DIET CHANGES: WHERE TO START

Food-based plans should provide adequate amounts of all nutrients except calories. Planning, as well as having a good knowledge base about foods, is crucial to success. Whether we count calories or not, food-based plans generally provide from 1,200 to 1,800 calories per day. It is important to divide your calories throughout the day, beginning with breakfast and including between-meal snacks. Eating a meal in the morning is important in order to bring your body out of its fasting mode, when you are burning fewer calories. Additionally, several pediatric studies appear to have found a relationship between eating breakfast and a decrease in the incidence of obesity. Clinical studies have shown that consuming fewer, larger meals is associated with increased body fat as opposed to eating smaller, more frequent meals providing the same amount of calories per day. And long periods of time between meals can create extreme

> *Food-based plans should provide adequate amounts of all nutrients except calories. Planning, as well as having a good knowledge base about foods, is crucial to success.*

hunger and lead to overeating during mealtime or eating inappropriate foods before the next meal is available.

Begin by planning to eat at least five servings of fruits and vegetables each day. Double your portion of vegetables at dinner and decrease the starch. Add fruit to your morning cereal and replace a high-calorie snack such as a candy bar with fresh veggies and lowfat dip. Seek lower-fat alternatives to foods you are currently consuming. For example, switch from whole milk to 1 percent or seek out lower-fat cheeses that are palatable to you. Change your cooking methods from frying to grilling, broiling, baking, and pan sautéing. Don't drink your calories. Avoid fruit drinks, sodas, and gourmet coffees loaded with fat and sugar. Increase your fiber intake by choosing whole grains and raw fruits and vegetables, as well as fiber-enriched cereals. Keep a record of the foods and beverages you are consuming each day. Make an effort to learn the calorie and fat content of foods using counter booklets and food labels. Gain an understanding of what an appropriate portion size is. Drink adequate amounts of fluid, especially water.

> *Studies have shown that consuming fewer, larger meals is associated with increased body fat as opposed to eating smaller, more frequent meals providing the same amount of calories per day.*

LONG-TERM SUCCESS

The word *diet* is from the Greek *diaita*, meaning literally "manner of living." This very connotation encourages us to see that losing and managing weight is dependent upon changes in the way we live our lives. The average dieter today usually has no difficulty entering into a weight-loss program (whether self-initiated or with professional guidance). Often the person has a clear goal in mind and has developed a plan (a particular diet or exercise program) to achieve that goal. But few recognize that winning the weight-loss battle is more than reaching the goal weight. Losing weight is probably the least difficult part of any weight-management plan, which is why so many people are successful at it. But many do not seem to recognize that losing weight does not solve the problem of obesity any more than taking one dose of insulin will cure diabetes.

> *Losing weight is probably the least difficult part of any weight-management plan, which is why so many people are successful at it. But many do not seem to recognize that losing weight does not solve the problem of obesity any more than taking one dose of insulin will cure diabetes.*

The evidence of this ability to repeatedly lose substantial amounts of weight with subsequent regain has become so prevalent in our society that we have a named it "yo-yo dieting," and we have become a nation of "chronic" dieters. What we have come to realize from this vicious cycle is that though weight loss can be difficult, maintaining weight loss is where the hard work comes in. Many people never recognize the need to plan this phase of their weight-management program and therefore are without the skills—which are different than the skills needed for weight loss—to maintain their loss. Often they return to their former eating habits or "food skills," the very ones which led to their prior state of obesity.

Maintenance

This leads us to a discussion of "maintenance diets." Let's begin by examining the habits of those who have been successful at maintaining their loss. The National Weight Control Registry (a database) keeps track of over 2,000 people who have successfully lost at least 30 pounds and have been able to maintain that loss for greater than 1 year.[8] The average participant in the study has lost over 60 pounds and has kept at least 30 pounds of it off for an average of 6 years. Similarly, nutritionist Anne Fletcher, author of *Thin for Life*, examined the daily eating habits of over 200 people who had lost an average of 64 pounds and maintained their loss for an average of 11 years.[9] Although we cannot call these results "permanent," they provide evidence that weight loss can be maintained and that chronic dieting is not the expectation for the overweight and the obese.

Several methods for prevention of regaining weight are evident among this population. Just because these people have lost their weight doesn't mean they are free to eat whatever they like. Maintaining the loss is a long-term, probably lifelong, endeavor. Most continue to watch what they're eating, choosing lowfat and fat-free foods as well as cooking without much fat or oil. According to the registry, these people maintain a lower energy intake, a self-reported average of 1,380 calories per day. Many continue to dine out two to three times per week (including fast food once a week), but they are cognizant of the foods they eat. Those tracked by Anne Fletcher describe their diets as "lowfat" and higher in fruits, vegetables, and whole grains. They also reported that they had accepted the fact that they couldn't go back to their old way of eating. Other activities found to be associated with maintaining weight loss include self-monitoring (getting on the scales) at least once a week and regular exercise (registry participants report burning an average of 2,800 calories per week).

Annual surveys of those in the National Weight Control Registry show that success is based on lifestyle changes such as the following:

- Eating less of certain types of foods (portion controlling)
- Counting calories (calorie awareness and maintaining a moderate calorie intake)
- Eating lower-fat foods and limiting fat intake to approximately 30 percent of calories or less
- A commitment to exercise, expending an average of 2,800 calories per week (equivalent to walking 3 to 4 miles per day)
- Monitoring weight at least once a week

The most encouraging piece of information to come out of the registry is that weight loss can be maintained and that there is a consensus on how to maintain it. What appears most evident to us is that there is a big distinction between losing weight and maintaining weight loss. It is also notable that permanent weight loss is a multifactorial endeavor and plans should encourage exercise and activity, as well as guidelines for addressing behaviors and developing strategies for change. Many programs are lacking in the behavioral-support area. Few programs address the "whys" of what we eat, leaving us open to failure after successfully losing weight. Seldom do many of us examine the reasons we eat or take a clear look at the stimuli that tell us we are hungry. There are physiological responses to the need for food, but more often we eat in response to external cues such as the smell or sight of food or the time of day. Many of us eat in response to our emotions or when we are bored or stressed. It may also be difficult for some of us to distinguish between the sensations of hunger and thirst. Many nutrition counselors recommend consuming a glass of water when we feel the need to snack to see if the sensation of hunger will diminish.

> *There are physiological responses to the need for food, but more often we eat in response to external cues such as the smell or sight of food or the time of day. Many of us eat in response to our emotions or when we are bored or stressed.*

The reasons for eating (other than hunger) are endless. Studies have shown we eat more when we are not getting enough sleep, using food to increase alertness (think of the "4 o'clock slump" at work). Foods are also symbolic to us and may take on a great deal of emotional meaning. Eating them rewards us with the good feelings we had when consuming them in the past. According to Anne Fletcher, a large percentage of obese people who struggle with weight are often eating for emotional reasons, whereas successful losers learn to get pleasure from other things in life.

THE IMPORTANCE OF EXERCISE

Multiple studies have shown a strong correlation between maintaining weight loss and exercising. Engaging in regular exercise or physical activity appears to be of paramount importance to maintaining a lower body weight. Current recommendations from the federal government are for approximately 30 minutes of exercise per day, seven times per week, for all adults.[10] In addition to structured exercise, it is also important to incorporate increased physical activity into your lifestyle. Small changes in daily routines (such as shunning the elevator in favor of the stairs) may afford us an increase in calorie expenditure that can add up to weight maintenance. An article by Susan Kayman and colleagues, published in the *American Journal of Clinical Nutrition*, examines weight-control behaviors among overweight women who either relapsed or maintained their loss.[11] Eighty-seven percent of the maintainers exercised, whereas none of the relapsers reported any increase in physical activity. And though the overall contribution to calorie deficit may be smaller than what can be achieved with dietary restriction, it is clear that exercise has a place in every weight-control program. Exercise may be more important for preventing the fall in resting metabolic rate that occurs with dieting, for improving flexibility, for maintaining or enhancing muscle mass, for improving cardiorespiratory endurance, and for increasing motor-skill performance. Physical activity has also been reported to decrease appetite and is related to improved emotional and psychological well-being, which are themselves important to successful weight maintenance.

And yet, exercise is one of those words, like *spinach* or *Brussels sprouts*, which is hard to hear without grimacing just a little. Sure, some of us like to exercise, just as some of us like Brussels sprouts. And whether we like them or not, we know that exercise and Brussels sprouts are both *good for us*. But as usual, the headline writers for the magazines we see in supermarket checkout aisles hit us where we really live. "Lose 30 Pounds Without Exercising," they may say, in the same appealing way that the very next magazine may declare: "New Diet Melts Fat While You Sleep."

But the energy equation is clear, and in our heads, if not in our hearts, we all know it. To lose weight and keep it off, we not only need to eat less, we need to move more. In fact, the key to maintaining weight loss seems to be in increasing our level of physical activity, along with eating less. Both sides of the equation are critical.

So maybe the key is not to think of *exercise*, which many of us will always associate with sit-ups and mile runs and jumping jacks under the stern gaze of a high school coach or physical education teacher. Maybe the key is to think of *playing*, a much more appealing concept that involves moving our bodies to have fun. This could include jogging, shooting basketball with our kids, going to a regular aerobics class after work, even simply taking a walk with a loved one after dinner—whatever we find relaxing, enjoyable, and mindless in a pleasurable way. But related to this is another important concept, that of *lifestyle changes*. In large and small ways, we have to look for daily opportunities to walk or cycle instead of drive. We have to choose the stairs over the elevator, the steps over the escalator, the far side of the parking lot over the 10-minute cruise to find the perfect parking space only feet from the mall entrance. We have to volunteer, again and again, for working up a little sweat and a faster heartbeat during our day-to-day lives. When this becomes second nature, not only will we be in better shape, we will also be much more capable of losing and managing weight. Not incidentally, we will manage stress better and, thus, from an emotional standpoint, we will have a higher degree of control over the psychological cues that trigger eating in the absence of hunger.

> *Maybe the key is to think of playing, a much more appealing concept that involves moving our bodies to have fun.*

"Imagine a new drug that could decrease stress, increase energy levels, improve sleep, decrease body fat and blood pressure, and improve levels of cholesterol," write a group of researchers from the National Institute for Fitness and Sport in Indianapolis. "Most individuals would rush to their physicians to get a prescription and would not hesitate to seek out a lifetime supply. Unfortunately, no such wonder drug exists; however, all of the physical and mental health benefits mentioned above are possible with a consistent program of regular physical activity, exercise, and proper nutrition."[12]

The flip side of the high proportion of American adults who are obese or overweight (three in five) is the low proportion of American adults who get the recommended minimum 30 minutes a day of physical activity—only one in five.

To get the first ratio down, we need to get the second ratio up. That's true for us as a nation, but also for each of us as an individual. So how to start?

Medical Exam

If you are over 45, or if you are under 45 but badly out of shape, it would be wise to see your doctor for a checkup before embarking on a vigorous exercise program. Particular danger signs that indicate you need a physical exam are growing weakness and fatigue, a history of fainting or dizziness, an increasing problem of breathlessness with exertion, chest pain, or heart palpitations. Recall our earlier discussion of masked problems that can underlie the condition of obesity. Problems to look out for can include heart disease, vascular disease, chronic lung disease, and diabetes. Of course, people with arthritis or other conditions affecting their bones and joints should also talk to their health-care provider and discuss their special needs before beginning an exercise program.

If you pass muster with your doctor, though, you're out of excuses. How do you get from where you are now to where you want to be?

Self-Assessment

Earlier in this chapter we discussed the notion of a food diary, or journal, in which you record everything you eat in the course of a day. Just the act of paying attention, over time, causes you to become more conscious of food, and more thoughtful in the way you prepare and eat your meals. The same can be true of exercise.

At the Johns Hopkins Weight Management Center, new clients are encouraged to chart a week of their physical activity by keeping exercise logs. Anyone who works in a law firm will be familiar with the concept of dividing a day into one-hour increments and tracking the number of minutes spent on various tasks within each hour. But you don't have to be a lawyer to play this game—and profit from it. For each hour in the day, record (or estimate) the time you spend in physical activity that is vigorous enough to cause an increase in heartbeat. The activity must last for 3 minutes or more to be counted. It could include everything from taking the stairs instead of the elevator to your office, to vacuuming or gardening, to playing your weekly game of squash. However, don't count just walking around your office or home to conduct normal daily activities.

Keep this log for a week. At the end of the week, count up the total minutes you have spent in vigorous physical activity. Then divide it by seven. That result is the average amount of time you devote each day to exercise—whether you think of it that way or not. If you spend 10 minutes a day or less doing anything that could qualify as exercise, you have fairly earned the dread label of "couch potato." On the other end of the scale, if you spend more than 40 minutes per day in exercise, you qualify in our society's terms as very active. Odds are you are somewhere in between. Furthermore, if you compare your result now to the result you would have gotten at age 15 or age 25, you will probably have to concede that you have grown less active with age.

That means that even as your metabolism has slowed with age (incidentally a not-inevitable concomitant of aging), you are compounding the whammy on your waistline by also cutting back on calorie-burning exercise. No wonder so many of us see the thickening we do as we move into our 30s, 40s and beyond.

Goals of Exercise

For people who are getting 10 minutes or less of exercise per day, and have received their doctor's green light, any increase in activity is bound to be beneficial. But if you are ready to swing for the fence, it is helpful to know more about various types of exercise and to understand that there is scientific agreement on how much and what types of exercise you must undertake in order to increase your level of physical fitness over time.

Target Heart Rate

First, it is important to understand what your *target heart rate* during exercise should be. You can measure your heart rate by counting your pulse rate as follows: Hold the fingertips of your three middle fingers against the side of your neck, where you can feel your carotid artery, or beside the tendon in the inside of your wrist for the radial artery. Once you detect your pulse, count the number of beats you feel in a 30-second period. Then multiply by two to get your heart rate per minute. An average heart rate for someone who does not work out regularly might be 70 or 80 beats per minute seated, at rest (the normal range is from 60 to 100 beats per minute at rest).

To calculate your target heart rate during exercise, begin by subtracting your age from 220. Thus, if you are 40 years old, you would subtract 40 from 220 and get 180. This figure is called your *maximum heart rate* in beats per minute. Then, subtract your resting heart rate (which you have already measured at, say 80) from your maximum heart rate (180) to get 100 beats per minute. This is the maximum increase

---

Heart-Rate Calculations

Resting Heart Rate = number of beats per minute while at rest

Maximum Heart Rate = 220 − your age

Target Heart Rate = [(maximum heart rate − resting heart rate) × 60%] + resting heart rate

over your resting heart rate that your heart, in theory, can achieve. Now, since it would not be safe to exercise at this extreme level (even for trained athletes) you are going to add only part of this theoretical limit to your resting heart rate to determine your target heart rate while exercising.

If you have been sedentary, multiply your theoretical maximum increase in heart rate over resting rate (100 beats per minute) by 60 percent—arriving at 60 beats per minute. Add your resting heart rate of 80 back in. Your target heart rate is 60 plus 80, or 140 beats per minute. If you are in better physical condition, multiply 100 by 70 percent, to reach 70. Add your resting heart rate of 80 back in. Your target heart rate is 70 plus 80, or 150 beats per minute.

To reach a higher level of physical fitness, you must regularly engage in some form of physical activity that will push your heart rate to your target heart rate zone for at least 20 to 30 minutes every other day—somewhere in that 140 to 150 zone, for example. Sound tough? It can be done. And once you begin hitting that mark regularly, don't be surprised if your body actually seems to crave a daily workout. As before, don't push yourself to the point of dizziness, nausea, tightness in your chest, or extreme breathlessness. If it takes you an unusual length of time to recover from small amounts of exercise, you should consult again with your doctor.

If your treadmill or other workout machine doesn't have an electronic gizmo to monitor your heart rate while you are using it, a simple measure is the "talk test"—if your heart is pounding too hard and your lungs are working too fast for you to talk comfortably, throttle back. You are not taking off in a sprint, you are embarking on a marathon that will last for the rest of your life—a life you are working on prolonging.

Consistent Exercise—Lasting Weight Control

As important as exercise is, it may be a little dismaying to find that calories and pounds do not magically melt away, even with a vigorous exercise program. This reflects the fact that weight is *much* easier to pack on in the first place than it is to lose. Also, without concomitant changes in eating behavior, the calories burned in exercise tend to be compensated for by increased food consumption. Thus, most studies show that it is unlikely that a program of exercise *alone* will result in more than a few pounds of weight loss. Nevertheless, there is no substitute for exercise in maintaining weight loss and physical fitness. Think of the tortoise who won the race with the hare by chugging along while the hare took a nap. You want to be the tortoise. Your success will be measured by heightened energy, a general increase in muscle tone and vigor, and by the fact that through a regular exercise program, you can keep off the pounds you lose by dieting.

> *Your success will be measured by heightened energy, a general increase in muscle tone and vigor, and by the fact that through a regular exercise program, you can keep off the pounds you lose by dieting.*

Many long-term dieters who are successful in maintaining weight loss have become religiously committed to walking. If you walk at a brisk pace (4.5 miles per hour, which is stepping out at a healthy pace), and if you weigh 200 pounds, it will take you 29 minutes to burn 200 calories. That means if you walk vigorously for an hour a day, you will burn 400 calories a day, or 2,800 calories a week. Recall that each pound of adipose tissue (fat) is roughly equivalent to 3,500 calories. You are "losing" the equivalent of four-fifths of a pound per week with a vigorous, hour-long daily walk. This may not sound like much on a daily or weekly basis, but it will add up to the equivalent of 40 pounds in a year! But the key is that it must be done *consistently*. We all know how devilishly hard that can turn out to be in practice. And it also must be done *together with* restraint in eating. If either half of the equation is neglected, it is a virtual certainty that you will not achieve your goal of lasting weight control. The actual amount of weight you lose, of course, will depend on how much more or less you eat when you increase your exercise level. Thus, if you overcompensate through your diet, you could actually gain weight while walking several miles a day.

For the sake of comparison, the average 200-pounder will burn 200 calories during:

- 53 minutes of sweeping floors
- 33 minutes of gardening
- 29 minutes of walking
- 22 minutes of bicycling
- 19 minutes of jogging
- 17 minutes of swimming laps
- 13 minutes of playing racquetball

A 100-pound person, ironically, must work at each activity about twice as long to burn the same number of calories. This reflects a simple law of physics. Only half the energy is required to move half the mass. The relative benefits of competitive or more active sports are obvious. At any weight, you burn calories much faster with a racquet in your hand than with a carpet sweeper. Yet to repeat, any degree of activity, including housework, will add up over time and is better than inactivity. In fact, it is quite possible to accumulate enough physical activity during the course of the day, by walking regularly and avoiding laborsaving devices, to equal or exceed the calories that are burned by an intensive half-hour workout at the gym. Even fidgeting and other under-appreciated forms of physical activity count. The person who paces out on the street while waiting for a table at a busy restaurant is burning many more calories than the person who is "lucky" enough to snare the empty seat at the front of the restaurant while waiting. Guess which person is most likely to retain more of those delicious calories after the dinner.

> *It is quite possible to accumulate enough physical activity during the course of the day, by walking regularly and avoiding laborsaving devices, to equal or exceed the calories that are burned by an intensive half-hour workout at the gym.*

Aerobic and Anaerobic Exercise

You may have heard exercises described as *aerobic* and *anaerobic*. Aerobic exercises cause your body to burn oxygen by accelerating your heart rate and breathing over a relatively long period of time. This includes activities such as aerobic dancing (hence the name), swimming, working out on a treadmill or stationary bicycle, or using a rowing machine—all relatively low-impact, joint-friendly activities that are recommended for most people. *Anaerobic* exercises—such as weight lifting—require short bursts of energy and do not accelerate your heart rate over an extended period of time. But they are also important. Weight-resistance training is vital for everyone, even for seniors, in order to maintain muscle tone and to strengthen bones. Both aerobic and anaerobic exercises should be a part of everyone's fitness program.

Warm Up and Cool Down

Finally, as the group of exercise and fitness specialists from Indianapolis point out, proper warming up and cooling down must be an integral part of anyone's exercise program. You should warm up with 5 to 10 minutes of very low-intensity exercise, followed by muscle stretching, and cool down in the same way until your heart rate falls below 100 beats per minute. This helps to avoid dizziness that can be caused by blood pooling in the arms and legs, and it also helps to minimize muscle soreness that can make it that much harder to start exercising the next time.[13]

The Roots of Motivation: How to Get Started and Stick with It

We have mentioned the important role that support groups play in helping people stay involved and committed to weight-loss programs. Knowing that you are accountable to others on a regular basis is invaluable in staying focused on your goals. The same is true for exercise. Many people find that having a commitment to meet an "exercise buddy" on a regular basis literally keeps them on track. On the other hand, there are several leading reasons that people frequently cite for failing to exercise regularly:

- Lack of time in one's daily schedule
- Lack of a convenient place or setting to exercise
- Lack of enjoyment in exercise
- Failure in past exercise programs

In view of the health benefits that can accrue from exercise, as well as the serious consequences of not exercising, most of these barriers reveal themselves to be thin excuses. But for many people, they are real barriers nevertheless. We need to work on knocking these excuses down, one by one. One technique that can be useful in addressing the number one excuse, lack of time, is to schedule exercise like any other important appointment. Another is to select activities that can be performed at home in what we call "double-time," such as pedaling an exercise bicycle while reading, listening to music, or watching television. This addresses lack of time, because no additional time is needed, and lack of convenient setting as well as lack of enjoyment, because you can do something else you find pleasurable while exercising in the comfort of your own home.

Some weight-control professionals have found that *pedometers* or *accelerometers*—tiny meters that clip on your belt and count steps or movement over the course of the day—are very helpful motivators, especially for individuals who are just getting into the swing of physical activity and need positive reinforcement. Researcher Kelly Brownell, director of the Yale Center for Eating and Weight Disorders, recommends an electronic pedometer that not only counts one's steps in walking or jogging, but also calculates the total distance traveled and the total number of calories burned. "This feedback can be highly rewarding and can be a constant reminder that any increase in your activity can be helpful," he writes.[14] (See appendix for more information on purchasing a pedometer.)

As for failure to succeed at sustaining increased physical activity, the past should be viewed as a learning experience. By conservatively planning a program that matches your lifestyle, broadening the definition of exercise to include walking and decreased use of laborsaving devices, and committing to monitor your activities by keeping a daily log, it should be much more likely that the past will be mere prelude, and the results most gratifying in terms of health and fitness, energy level, and weight control.

Behavioral Issues

Just as a multidisciplinary approach to weight loss has been shown to be effective, so, too, is this approach for weight maintenance. We have looked at dietary interventions and the importance of exercise. Let's take a look at the behavioral issues involved. The root of behavioral success starts in the active phase of weight loss as we begin to make the changes that will help us to reach our goal. Those who are successful at losing and maintaining their loss are able to devise personal strategies and develop internal sources. According to Kayman, important behaviors include seeking social support (talking), either from friends and family or from a professional setting, as well as learning to problem solve (confronting problems) and to develop coping mechanisms (seeking solutions). Relapsers tended to use escape and avoidance, such as alcohol and medication, when problems arose. Self-monitoring techniques also seem to be related to success and include keeping food logs and weighing yourself on a regular basis.

> *Hunger awareness is an important skill to master. Many of us do not take the time to determine when we are truly hungry as opposed to eating from boredom, anxiety, and stress or emotional pain.*

Hunger awareness is an important skill to master. Many of us do not take the time to determine when we are truly hungry as opposed to eating from boredom, anxiety, and stress or emotional pain. True hunger may be different for all of us and only you can determine whether or not it is time to eat. Consider tracking times and events surrounding your intake in your food log. This will help you determine what some of your triggers to eat may be. The following are guidelines to help you learn whether you need to fuel your body or gain control of unhealthful eating.

Consider the time. When did you last eat? If you have eaten a substantial meal within the past 3 to 4 hours, chances are you are not hungry.

Consider the trigger. Was it external, such as a sensory (sight and smell) stimulus? Did someone talk to you about food? Did you pass a fast-food restaurant on the road? Was it internal, such as stress to complete the day's assignments or feeling upset over family tensions?

Consider the event. Are you at a meeting with food? Are you attending a social event? Are you eating simply because the food is available?

These are just a few examples. As you begin to see how you are eating in unhealthy ways, consider the following strategies.

Have a plan for the day. Include three meals and a couple of snacks that fit within your calorie budget.

Separate yourself from triggers. Consider an alternative behavior to distract your thoughts about eating.

Wait it out. Have a large glass of water or a calorie-free beverage and wait 20 to 30 minutes to see if the desire passes.

Avoid the stimulus. For example, consider avoiding the vending area and removing tempting foods from your home.

Substitute. Consider a "fun-size" candy bar in place of a full size and remember to budget the calories in your daily allotment.

Old habits, such as eating while reading or watching television, must be broken and strategies for eating appropriately at social functions must be developed. As much as we like to eat, we are often eating without any thought about what is in our mouth. How often do we sit in front of the TV and consume an entire bag of chips without realizing it? Or attend a party and sit down in front of the peanut bowl, only to consume the entire container while chatting with a friend? This is referred to as "mindless eating," when we fail to take the time to think about and enjoy the foods we are eating.

Awareness is the first step toward breaking these unhealthy habits. Make an agreement with yourself to enjoy your food. Consider eating as a solo activity, meaning you will not eat and drive, nor eat and study, nor eat and watch TV. Eat slowly and savor the activity and flavors involved in each bite. When at a party, station yourself away from the foods so you are not tempted to grab before you think and munch without the realization that you are eating.

Last but not least, it is also important to overcome negative self-talk and build an inner vocabulary that promotes a healthy response to setbacks and perceived failures. It is rare to find people who have not encountered times when they ate more food than they should, or who have not eaten foods and beverages that are excessive in calories. For those who are attempting to lose weight, these events can trigger thoughts of failure and disappointment, which in turn, may lead to overeating for an extended period of time or the abandonment of any dietary program. It is so easy to tell ourselves, "You might as well give up. You're never going to be able to lose weight." Recognizing and addressing our negative "self-talk" is a valuable skill that enables us to recover from occasional lapses on our weight-loss journey. Drs. G. Alan Marlatt and Judith Gordon write in their book, *Relapse Prevention*, that recovery from lapses can occur by following a few simple steps:

> Recognizing and addressing our negative "self-talk" is a valuable skill that enables us to recover from occasional lapses on our weight-loss journey.

- Recognize and stop what you are doing.
- Stay calm. Don't succumb to blaming yourself and feeling out of control. Remind yourself that a lapse is a single event and not a lifestyle.

- Review your previous success and remind yourself of your goals.
- Learn from the situation. Consider why this happened.
- Take charge. Change your immediate behavior, which may mean leaving the environment that caused you to eat inappropriately.[15]

As this chapter illustrates, a comprehensive approach to weight control, one which encompasses the key components of diet, behavior, and physical activity, is essential to achieve, and more importantly still, to maintain, optimal weight control.

CHAPTER 4

Drug Treatment for Weight Loss

One pill makes you larger
And one pill makes you small,
And the ones that mother gives you
Don't do anything at all.

—GRACE SLICK, "WHITE RABBIT"

WHEN IT COMES to health, we Americans are an impatient people. We like to fix things, the quicker the better. Once-dreaded scourges such as typhoid, pneumonia, and polio are all much smaller threats to our health because of drugs or vaccines developed in the past 50 years.

Shots are okay in a pinch, but pills are our preferred mode of administration. So the question suggests itself logically: Why can't science invent drugs that we can take—possibly with a shot, but preferably by mouth—to "fix" obesity? Why can't we all be like Alice in the song by Jefferson Airplane? Pop a pill and get smaller overnight—by at least a few dress sizes?

Indeed, if we can believe the ads in the magazines we pick up at the supermarket checkout line, don't we have drugs and other products like this already?

The short answer is *No*. But that has not stopped many from trying. The field of weight reduction has as checkered a history as any branch of medicine. For most of the past century, scientists and hucksters alike have searched for that magic elixir that will keep us slim and trim without exertion, willpower, or sweat. So far, it's as elusive as the

---

Fat-Fighting Treatments That Failed: A Century of Disappointments

For more than 100 years, hopes have been raised and dashed by plausible-sounding anti-obesity treatments that ended up doing more harm than good. This has been a persistent refrain in medicine, reflecting both the dimensions of the overweight problem, and the extreme complexity of trying to modify appetite and digestion.

Date	Drug	Negative Outcome
1893	Thyroid	Hyperthyroidism
1934	Dinitrophenol	Cataracts and neuropathy (peripheral nerve damage)
1937	Amphetamine	Addiction
1967	"Rainbow pills" (digitalis; diuretics)	Deaths
1971	Aminorex	Pulmonary hypertension
1978	Collagen-based Very Low Calorie Diet	Deaths
1997	Fenfluramine (the "fen" part of fen-phen)	Valvular insufficiency (heart-valve damage); primary pulmonary hypertension

---

Source: Adpated from G. A. Bray and F. L. Greenway, "Current and Potential Drugs for Treatment of Obesity," *Endocrine Review* 20, no. 6 (1999).

fabled silver mines of El Dorado. (See sidebar, "Fat-Fighting Treatments That Failed.")

It is possible that in the next decade or two, fundamental discoveries about genetics, hormones, and neurotransmitters—the chemicals that mediate communication between the brain and organs such as muscles, intestines, and the stomach—may lead to some truly effective advances. Pharmaceutical companies are looking with renewed interest at the possibility of creating new types of anti-obesity drugs. Their focus on this objective has been sharpened by two important trends—the increasing understanding of obesity as a chronic condition that might be treatable in a way analogous to diabetes or hypertension, and fundamental advances in molecular biology that are leading to new insights in the relation between brain, body, and behavior.[1] But the release of new drugs, even if researchers' fondest hopes are realized sometime this century, will not happen soon enough to bring relief to anyone who needs to lose weight *now*, whether to drop inches around the waist for an upcoming class reunion, or to moderate the dangerous symptoms of type 2 diabetes or sleep apnea.

Nevertheless, and fortunately, there are some helpful drugs that weight-management professionals do prescribe as *adjuncts* to supervised programs of weight reduction. Think of them as boosters. These drugs produce modest weight loss for limited periods of time. They enhance the good work we do for ourselves through low-calorie diets and exercise programs. However, most of these drugs cannot be taken indefinitely and tend to become less effective over time (that is, typically weight is later regained even when the drug continues to be taken). Thus, they produce lasting effects only if our new habits of diet and exercise persist after the drugs themselves are begun.

Where have we heard that before?

> *It is possible that in the next decade or two, fundamental discoveries about genetics, hormones, and neurotransmitters—the chemicals that mediate communication between the brain and organs such as muscles, intestines, and the stomach—may lead to some truly effective advances.*

HOW DO WEIGHT-REDUCTION DRUGS WORK?

Although there are some compounds that work by more than one mechanism, drugs used for weight control fall into the following three main categories.

Appetite Suppressants

Some medications have the effect of reducing our normal degree of appetite. They do this chiefly by inhibiting the brain cells' absorption (or reuptake) of certain neurotransmitters, such as serotonin and norepinephrine, whose creation is part of a feedback loop that causes a feeling of satisfaction as we eat. The effect of modifying this chemical process is the creation of a feeling of satiety, or a sensation of fullness, without having to eat as much food as would otherwise be required. Some of these drugs also have a stimulant effect on the central nervous system, meaning that we will burn calories faster.

Stimulants

Some drugs act on our central nervous system to speed up our metabolisms (the rate at which we burn calories even while resting). They are called *thermogenic*. Because we burn more calories when using such a drug, there is less "excess" energy remaining to store in our adipose tissues. Hence less fat is created for every unit of food we eat in excess of our usual (pre-drug) daily energy needs.

The classic examples of stimulant appetite suppressants are the amphetamines. One nonprescription drug of this type is nicotine (thus the persistent, unhealthy association between smoking and thinness). The combination of caffeine and ephedrine, which are available separately over the counter without a doctor's prescription, also falls into this category. Although widely used as a component of a variety of nonprescription appetite-suppressing medicines, ephedra (the parent form of ephedrine, marketed frequently by its Chinese name *ma huang* in herbal medicines) can cause many side effects and is surrounded by growing controversy related to its reported propensity to increase the risk of cardiac events and strokes, especially in people who have underlying cardiac disease. Taken as diet pills, neither ephedra compounds nor caffeine are recommended by most doctors. We shall discuss the nonprescription drugs separately from the prescription drugs.

Fat Blockers

Much research and development activity by the major pharmaceutical companies has focused on drugs that will prevent digestion of the fat in the foods we eat. One recently approved drug, orlistat (Xenical), interferes with the digestion of some of the fat that we eat. It binds to and thus blocks the action of certain of the enzymes that are needed to break down dietary fats into their component fatty acids, whisking them through the intestines and out of the body before they can be absorbed into the bloodstream. Obviously this kind of drug cannot save us from sweet or starchy junk diets, but it comes on like gangbusters against the waist-padding fat in dairy products, potato chips, fried chicken, and other hard-to-resist fast-food favorites.

WHAT PRESCRIPTION DRUGS ARE AVAILABLE?

Currently, the list is a fairly short one. The most important existing drugs are summarized in table 5. In general, most prescription drugs approved for weight control work by suppressing appetite—that is, they modify brain chemistry in subtle ways to make us feel satisfied from eating smaller amounts of food. Studies of patients taking these drugs have shown that patients reduce food intake compared to patients taking placebos (inert substances). Other drugs that fall in this category, but which are currently less commonly prescribed than those listed in table 5, are mazindol (Mazanor, Sanorex) and diethylpropion (Tenuate).

Although amphetamines are technically—and legally—available, they are rarely if ever prescribed any more for weight control because of the abuse and addiction problems that very often accompanied their use.

In addition to the drugs approved specifically for weight control, there are other drugs developed primarily to treat other diseases or conditions, which have the effect of reducing appetite or weight. Doctors may prescribe them for weight-control purposes. This is known as an "off-label" use. Currently, there is some interest in the weight-reduction potential of the drug bupropion (Wellbutrin or Zyban), an antidepressant that is frequently prescribed to help people stop smoking. In a recent randomized, controlled study involving 50 women, the group on bupropion achieved an average weight loss of 4.9 percent at 8 weeks as compared with 1.3 percent for those on a placebo. A subset who stayed on bupropion for 24 weeks achieved an average weight loss of 12.9 percent.[2] Another drug that has been used by some doctors for weight reduction is fluoxetine (Prozac), a selective serotonin-reuptake inhibitor that is used primarily for the treatment of depression and obsessive-compulsive disorder. It may also be prescribed for bulimia nervosa, an eating disorder.[3] However, fluoxetine has not been shown to result in consistent or lasting weight loss, and can even be associated with weight gain instead of weight reduction. In general, we feel that it is unwise to use medicines for weight control that were developed, tested, and approved by the FDA for another purpose. It is precisely because these drugs have not been scientifically studied and tested for effectiveness and safety for the new use (weight control) that we do not recommend that you become one of the test subjects in an uncontrolled experiment, even if you are tempted and your physician can be persuaded to prescribe the drug off label. If any off-label use is truly effective and safe, you can be assured that the manufacturer will have a strong incentive to seek FDA approval for this new use for its drug.

> *Most prescription drugs approved for weight control work by suppressing appetite—that is, they modify brain chemistry in subtle ways to make us feel satisfied from eating smaller amounts of food.*

Table 5. Prescription Weight-Control Drugs Currently Approved by the FDA

Generic Name	Brand Name	How It Works	Daily Cost
Phentermine	Adipex-P, Fastin, Ionamin, Oby-trim	Suppresses appetite	15–30 milligrams per day in 1 or 2 doses: $1.03
Sibutramine	Meridia	Suppresses appetite; may also speed up metabolism	5, 10, or 15 milligrams per day in 1 daily dose: $2.99
Xenical	Orlistat	Inhibits digestion of fat	360 milligrams per day (if a person eats 3 meals per day); dose is 120 milligrams with each "high-fat meal": $3.96

WHEN IS DRUG THERAPY RECOMMENDED?

Prescription anti-obesity drugs are recommended only for people who are obese—that is, for those who have a BMI of 30 or above (see chapter 2), or those who have a BMI of 27 or above with significant weight-related diseases (comorbidities) such as high cholesterol, hypertension, or type 2 diabetes. In addition, anti-obesity drugs are recommended only for those who have tried and failed to lose weight through diet and exercise alone. These cautions are necessary because weight-reduction drugs, like all pharmaceutical agents, have a not-insignificant list of potential side effects. We will discuss the side effects a little later. In addition, prescription anti-obesity drugs are recommended for use *only* as part of a medically supervised program of dieting and exercise. Your doctor should periodically monitor their safety and effectiveness for as long as you are on them. Anti-obesity drugs are not the equivalent of a dose of penicillin, which will stop a bacterial infection in its tracks without a scintilla of conscious effort from us—indeed, while we lie groaning in bed. Obesity-fighting drugs work only with our active cooperation and help. They will only produce permanent changes if we summon the willingness and the discipline to make changes in our behavior, including the way we eat and the amount of physical activity we engage in. The drug that would safely allow us to wash down a box of chocolate chip cookies with a quart of whole milk and top it off with a pint of Ben and Jerry's—all without adding so much as a millimeter to our hips—has not been invented and likely never will be. In any event, that's not what doctors have at their disposal now.

> *Prescription anti-obesity drugs are recommended only for people who are obese—that is, for those who have a BMI of 30 or above, or those who have a BMI of 27 or above with significant weight-related diseases.*

A further caveat here: Anti-obesity drugs should be used only because someone needs to lose weight for medical reasons—not because they want to slim down a few pounds for cosmetic purposes.[4] Unfortunately, there is abundant evidence showing that medications are being overprescribed for some patients in this area as in other branches of medicine, a reminder of the incredible pressure felt by many to be slender and the pressure that patients are able to exert on physicians to give them the drugs they want.

A national telephone survey of more than 139,000 adults taken by the Centers for Disease Control and Prevention estimated that 4.6 million Americans, or 1 out of every 40 adults, had taken prescription drugs for weight loss in the 2-year period from 1996 to 1998. Women were nearly five times more likely to use them than were men (4 percent versus 0.9 percent), and among the ethnic groups in the survey, Hispanics had the highest rate of overall use (3.2 percent). Perhaps most troubling, though, was the fact that about one-quarter of those who had taken prescription drugs for weight loss did not meet the minimum criterion in that they did not have a BMI of 27 or above, based on their self-reported height and weight. This suggests that weight-loss medications "may be inappropriately used, especially among women, white persons, and Hispanic persons," said the researchers.[5]

It is possible that we are living in a watershed era, from a historical perspective, in that anti-obesity drugs may soon be prescribed for long-term, even chronic use, similar to statins for high cholesterol or ACE inhibitors for high blood pressure. Historically, few anti-obesity drugs have been tested for periods longer than 1 year. When they have been withdrawn, and patients have, in most cases, relapsed to something near their pre-study weight, these drugs have been regarded as a failure. However, in the new perspective that is coming to dominate the field of weight control, it makes sense that *no* drugs should be depended on to cure obesity. Rather, they should be regarded as simply one more contributor to the major change in dietary patterns and physical activity that alone will achieve lasting weight reduction.

> *It is possible that we are living in a watershed era, from a historical perspective, in that anti-obesity drugs may soon be prescribed for long-term, even chronic use, similar to statins for high cholesterol or ACE inhibitors for high blood pressure.*

WHAT ARE THE LIMITATIONS AND RISKS OF DRUG THERAPY?

Although anti-obesity drugs have a valid role in attacking obesity in those who are severely obese or who have medical problems associated with their obesity, they are crutches designed for temporary use, not as replacement limbs. Most of the time, weight loss achieved by these drugs levels off in 4 to 6 months, and then weight is slowly and steadily regained, whether the drug is continued or not.[6]

Considering that appetite suppressants are powerful agents and that all but orlistat act directly on brain chemistry to achieve their effects, it is not surprising, perhaps, that all, including orlistat, have a long list of potential side effects that patients and their doctors must be alert to. If your doctor prescribes an appetite suppressant (or any other drug), you should ask your doctor or pharmacist about potential side effects as well as the promised result. In addition, you should read carefully the patient information handout you will get with your prescription and take advantage of any patient-support program that is offered by the manufacturer for people taking their drug. (Such programs are currently offered by the makers of orlistat [Xenical], and by the makers of sibutramine [Meridia].)

> Although anti-obesity drugs have a valid role in attacking obesity in those who are severely obese or who have medical problems associated with their obesity, they are crutches designed for temporary use, not as replacement limbs.

In general, appetite suppressants have side effects such as insomnia, dry mouth, headache, nervousness, and constipation. In addition, sibutramine raises blood pressure and heart rate and thus may not be suitable for people with a history of stroke, heart disease, or uncontrolled high blood pressure. Also, doctors will want to know if you have ever suffered from alcohol or drug abuse, eating disorders, depression, migraines, glaucoma, or diabetes. Appetite suppressants are not usually appropriate for women who are pregnant or breast-feeding.[7]

Dexfenfluramine and fenfluramine, the two leading appetite suppressants that were both withdrawn from the market in 1997, were linked to a heightened risk of a rare and often fatal condition called *primary pulmonary hypertension*. Although it is believed that none of the existing appetite suppressants cause this disorder, which has a 45 percent fatality rate within 4 years, patients who are taking appetite suppressants should notify their doctors promptly if they notice chest pain, shortness of breath, a feeling of faintness, or swelling in their feet and ankles. Summarizing the existing literature, the NIH's Weight-Control Information Network says there have been "only a few" reports of primary pulmonary hypertension in people taking phentermine alone, and no reported cases with sibutramine.

Orlistat (Xenical), which works by blocking the absorption of up to 30 percent of dietary fat, has a different set of side effects to worry about, including urgent bowel movements, more frequent bowel movements, gas, and oily spotting. These side effects are the natural consequence of so much dietary fat passing undigested through the bowel. However, these issues have resolved for most patients in long-term trials.[8] Because orlistat blocks the digestion of fats, people taking it must supplement their diets with a multivitamin containing extra amounts of the fat-soluble vitamins—D, E, K, and beta-carotene.

WHAT ARE THE BENEFITS AND ADVANTAGES OF DRUG THERAPY?

Although the benefits of anti-obesity drugs may seem modest compared with the dramatic gains associated with weight-reduction surgery, they are, in fact, potentially important. There is a growing acknowledgment that for many obese people, even those who are seriously obese, weight reductions in the area of 5 to 15 percent are both realistically achievable and worthwhile in terms of securing better health. The best of the currently available prescription drugs, used in conjunction with dietary and lifestyle changes, can help achieve and sustain that kind of moderate reduction in weight.

A recent review of all published long-term studies of the leading anti-obesity drugs found that they have, overall, achieved results in the 5 to 15 percent range. Researcher Gary Glazer of the University of Rochester summarized all trials since 1960 comparing people on anti-obesity drugs with a control group on a placebo for periods of 36 weeks or greater as follows:

- Weight loss on phentermine was 8.1 percent, or 7.9 kilograms (17.4 pounds), in excess of weight loss achieved on a placebo.

> *There is a growing acknowledgment that for many obese people, even those who are seriously obese, weight reductions in the area of 5 to 15 percent are both realistically achievable and worthwhile in terms of securing better health.*

- Weight loss on sibutramine was 5 percent, or 4.3 kilograms (9.5 pounds), in excess of weight loss achieved on a placebo.
- Weight loss on orlistat was 3.4 percent, or 3.4 kilograms (7.5 pounds), in excess of weight loss achieved on a placebo.[9]

Historically, most anti-obesity drugs have been recommended and approved only for short-term use. However, as new drugs are developed, the medical profession is moving toward a change in perspective in which obesity may be treated with drugs (and complementary approaches) as a chronic condition over a period of years as opposed to weeks or months. This has been demonstrated in controlled trials of orlistat (Xenical), the fat-blocking digestion inhibitor, and of sibutramine (Meridia), the newest of the appetite suppressants.

Most anti-obesity drugs have been recommended and approved only for short-term use. However, as new drugs are developed, the medical profession is moving toward a change in perspective in which obesity may be treated with drugs (and complementary approaches) as a chronic condition over a period of years as opposed to weeks or months.

A recently completed long-term study called STORM (Sibutramine Trial of Obesity Reduction and Maintenance) found that in some individuals, sibutramine (Meridia), after it completes its original mission of reducing weight, can be effective for an additional 18 months in helping to keep the lost weight off. As all dieters know, it often proves easier to take pounds off in the first place than it is to keep them off afterward. In STORM, a group of 605 obese patients (with BMIs ranging from 30 to 45) were recruited by eight obesity centers in Europe to engage in a 6-month period of weight loss during which they took sibutramine and maintained a low-calorie diet. Three-quarters of the patients achieved a weight loss of 5 percent or more. These successful patients were then divided into two subgroups. One group continued to take sibutramine. Another group was switched (without its knowledge) to a placebo. Over the ensuing year and a half, four out of ten people on sibutramine were able to maintain at least 80 percent of their initial weight loss, whereas fewer than one out of six people on the placebo were able to maintain a comparable reduction. (However, it is also important to note that half of the placebo group and 42 percent of the sibutramine group dropped out during the year-and-a-half follow-up period, a not-unusual occurrence in long-term weight-loss trials.)

Perhaps most encouraging from a medical standpoint, were the noteworthy decreases in some of the most damaging indicators associated with obesity. Along with their weight reduction, patients experienced significant reductions in overall cholesterol, as well as in very-low-density-lipoprotein cholesterol (the most damaging kind), insulin, triglycerides, and other markers. In the second year, both groups, even the one on the placebo, experienced increases in their high-density-lipoprotein ("good") cholesterol counts. On the minus side, researchers noted that sibutramine resulted in increases in blood pressure and pulse rate.[10]

In a *British Medical Journal* editorial on the STORM study, Canadian researcher Jean-Pierre Després noted some of the limitations of the study as well as the areas of new possibilities it represents.[11] First he noted that, because the study was conducted at sophisticated clinics where a changing diet could be calibrated to the metabolic rate of participants, it is unlikely ordinary doctors can duplicate these results in the field. Second, by design, only those who responded well to sibutramine continued on to the second, 18-month part of the study. (Of the original 605 people, 138 were left behind at this point.) And third, more than 80 percent of the participants were women, as is typical of the general population seeking treatment for obesity. This despite the fact, as he said, that "men are generally characterized by a more dangerous form of obesity—visceral, or abdominal obesity"—in other words, the characteristic apple shape of men as opposed to the pear shape of women that was discussed in chapter 1. Therefore, he concluded, the STORM trial may open the door to future trials of anti-obesity drugs that would be targeted specifically at abdominally obese men with high coronary risk.

But, Després says, because sibutramine raises blood pressure and heart rate, this specific drug may turn out to be best suited only for insulin-resistant obese people with high blood lipids who do *not* suffer from high blood pressure—illustrating the level of complexity doctors and drug designers will have to pick their way through in search of drugs that can be taken safely, and effectively, for years on end.

DRUGS AS AN ADJUNCT TO THERAPY

One invariable, and regrettable, consequence of finding a successful new weight-loss drug is that consumers turn to it as the easy, unique

Fen-Phen: The Exotic-Sounding Heartbreaker

Sometimes if a medical treatment sounds too good to be true, it is. But hopes were high in the case of the diet-drug combination known as "fen-phen"—fenfluramine (Pondimin) and phentermine. Sales of these drugs and a related drug, dexfenfluramine (Redux), soared in the mid-1990s as doctors and patients alike thought that medical science, at long last, had hit pay dirt in the search for a safe, effective, fast-acting diet drug.

For a few years, Pondimin and Redux were one of the most spectacular success stories in the history of pharmaceuticals. In 1992, there had been 60,000 prescriptions written for fenfluramine. By 1997, more than 10 million prescriptions had been written for the "fen-phen" combination.[12]

The drugs' use in the combination known as "fen-phen" was spurred by a 1992 study showing an average weight loss of more than 31 pounds, or nearly 16 percent of body weight, in a group taking them for 34 weeks. "Dry mouth" was reported to be the most common side effect. Follow-up studies reported the weight loss was maintained for up to 3½ years as use of fen-phen continued.

key to their overweight problem. No single drug can be that key. The drugs we are discussing here are all prescription drugs, but determined patients are often able to get a beleaguered doctor—whether their own, or someone else's—to write them a prescription if they want a drug badly enough. Drug companies as well as other for-profit businesses understand this and have devoted millions of dollars to direct-to-consumer advertising, bypassing physicians entirely. Without question, that kind of promotion helped to fuel the fen-phen craze (see sidebar).[13]

Now we may see some of the same enthusiasm with regard to sibutramine (Meridia) and orlistat (Xenical), both of which are modestly effective over a long period of time. Leading figures in the scientific

---

The bandwagon came to a screeching halt shortly after doctors at the Mayo Clinic in Rochester, Minnesota, reported in 1997 that they had identified 24 cases of women with unusual heart-valve disease, similar to that seen in rare cases of a tumor called carcinoid or following ergotamine poisoning. Five of the women required heart-valve replacement. Eight developed pulmonary hypertension, a life-threatening disorder. All had been taking fen-phen for periods ranging from 5 to 19 months (averaging 1 year). The women ranged in age from 36 to 52 (averaging 44).[14]

When more such cases surfaced around the country—some involving patients who were taking only dexfenfluramine or fenfluramine individually—the FDA requested the withdrawal of those drugs from the market. Follow-up studies estimated that 23 percent to one-third of those taking dexfenfluramine or fenfluramine had cardiac-valve abnormalities.[15] However, a larger study of nearly 9,000 users of dexfenfluramine or fenfluramine found only 8 with clinically significant valve damage.[16]

Phentermine, which composed one-half of the "fen-phen" combination was not found to cause heart damage when taken alone, and it remains on the market as a prescription-only appetite suppressant.

understanding and treatment of obesity have cautioned us to remember that fixation on a drug solution would be a mistake. At best, drugs are an adjunct—an aid to achieving the healthy effects of changes in diet, eating patterns, and exercise that we must make to secure a lower weight for the long haul.

Illustrating this point, researchers from the University of Pennsylvania recently published results from a study they conducted of 53 obese women who were assigned randomly into three groups:

- The first group took sibutramine and were assigned a suggested diet and exercise schedule, but were not monitored as to compliance (drug-alone group).
- The second group took sibutramine and were assigned the same diet and exercise schedule as the first group, but they also underwent lifestyle modification by attending first weekly, then monthly, group sessions conducted by psychologists (drug-plus-lifestyle group).
- The third group took sibutramine, plus the lifestyle modification, plus they were put on an even stricter prescribed diet, consisting of 1,000 portion-controlled calories a day for the first 4 months (combined-treatment group).

One invariable, and regrettable, consequence of finding a successful new weight-loss drug is that consumers turn to it as the easy, unique key to their overweight problem. No single drug can be that key.

At the beginning of the experiment, women in all three groups were surveyed as to their expectations for weight loss. They all had high hopes—not untypical for those entering weight-loss treatment. Despite an average BMI of 37.7 (ranging from 34.1 to 41.3), putting all of them well into the obese category, they expected to lose an average of 25 percent of their initial body weight.

At the end of a year, the results were telling. The first group (drug alone) lost an average of 4.1 percent. The second group (drug-plus-lifestyle) lost an average of 10.8 percent. The third group (combined treatment) lost an average of 16.5 percent (see figure 4.1). And guess which group was most satisfied with the results!

"Our findings clearly showed that group lifestyle modification improved the pharmacologic treatment of obesity," the researchers wrote.[17] "We, like others, believe that lifestyle modification provides obese people strategies to manage the external food environment. These strategies include shopping from a list, storing foods out of sight, controlling portion sizes, avoiding fast-food restaurants, and keeping food records. By contrast, centrally acting weight loss medications, including sibutramine, seem to modify the internal environment by increasing satiation or by decreasing hunger or preoccupation with food."

Worth noting is that this study did not include a group of patients that got intensive diet and lifestyle therapy, but a placebo instead of an active drug. Though it is risky to make predictions, it is likely—based on the results of other studies—that this group would also have achieved substantial weight loss, possibly no less than that achieved with a drug. Other studies have demonstrated that a very important factor in achieving and sustaining weight loss is the intensity of the treatment provided—more frequent treatment visits, for example, are more

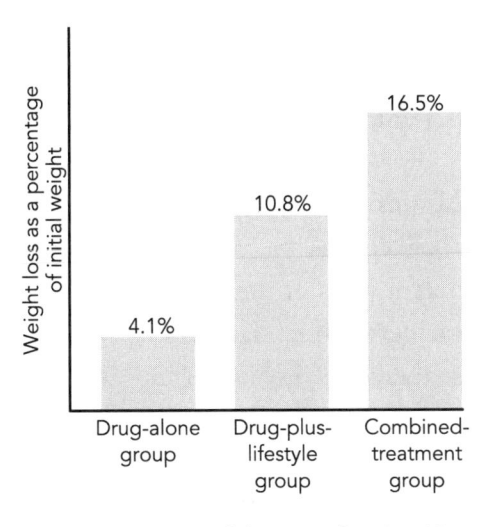

Figure 4.1—*Weight Loss After One Year*

effective than less frequent visits, even when the diet and other features of the programs are the same.

SUMMARY

The history of weight-reduction drugs is as checkered as the term "diet pills" might suggest. The road has been marked by many failures and some catastrophes, such as the fen-phen enthusiasm that resulted in heart damage to an alarming number of young, basically healthy women. However, a small armamentarium of FDA-approved prescription drugs is available to doctors. One new appetite suppressant (sibutramine), and the first inhibitor of fat digestion (orlistat), have been approved since 1997. More drugs are in the works as pharmaceutical companies continue their efforts on a wide front. They are spurred on by a new outlook whereby obesity is considered more akin to a chronic medical condition, like the diabetes it often engenders, than to a psychological failure of will and discipline. Because of this new perspective, there is increasing interest in finding medications that are safe and effective over a period of years instead of weeks. Nevertheless, it is unlikely that drugs by themselves will ever be able to reverse obesity. At best, they can reinforce diet and behavior programs, helping overweight people to develop new patterns of eating and exercise that must be maintained on a lifelong basis to be successful. Further, it is likely that only combinations of more than one drug, acting on different parts of the appetite and weight-control system, will be able to achieve substantial, consistent, and sustained weight loss. That is because there is a very powerful system of checks and balances built into this very important matter of ensuring that human beings do not lose weight. It is obvious that, throughout the ages, there was a survival benefit to being able to gain weight easily, and a penalty

> *The challenge for future drug treatment of obesity is to achieve control of multiple levels of our body's weight-defense mechanisms while minimizing side effects and toxicity.*

for those who were thin or had trouble gaining weight. (Which type of person would be most likely to make it through the winter or other times of food shortage?)

Given our biologically and genetically dictated preference for weight gain over weight loss, the proliferation of inexpensive, high-calorie, high-fat foods, along with the death of regular physical activity or labor for most adults is a recipe for disaster. The fact that we are unlikely to overcome our body's fail-safes unless we use multiple drugs to disable each of them is yet another consequence of the powerful physiologic mechanisms that act to avoid weight loss at all costs. Unfortunately, as exemplified by the problems we had with fen-phen, using more than one drug increases the chances of problems.

The challenge for future drug treatment of obesity is to achieve control of multiple levels of our body's weight-defense mechanisms while minimizing side effects and toxicity. It is a tall order, but we are making strides in the right direction as we learn more and more about the basic science and genetics of weight regulation.

CHAPTER 5

Surgery
Last Chance or Best Prospect?

OUR SURVEY OF treatments for obesity continues with perhaps the most radical choice—surgery. Obesity surgery—also called *bariatric* surgery, from the Greek *baros* (weight) and *iatrike* (medicine, surgery)—uses a variety of techniques to alter the normal passage of food into the stomach and through the small intestine. Because the size of the stomach is literally reduced, or a segment of the small intestine is bypassed, the obese person cannot eat the same volume of food in any given period of time as he or she could prior to the surgery. Attempts to eat too much too quickly result in vomiting or other unpleasant forms of feedback from the shortened digestive canal. In some procedures, diminishing the length of intestine that food passes through also diminishes the amount of nutrients absorbed by the body.

Although it can be defeated by an uncooperative patient, antiobesity surgery offers the motivated individual a clean break from past behavior patterns and a powerful tool to achieve consumption of less calories and, therefore, permanent weight loss.

This is a choice of last resort. It involves permanent changes to the body's own plumbing system and carries substantial risks. Patients must be carefully selected and must agree to modify their diets and eating patterns for the rest of their lives. Complications can require repeat surgery. Understandably, it is scary to contemplate. Bariatric surgery centers report overall mortality rates ranging from 0.5 percent (or less) to 1 or 2 percent. How many of us would go for a cruise on an ocean liner if we knew that one out of every hundred vessels leaving the dock never returned? We might do so, under duress, if the ship represented our only hope of escaping from a desperate situation—a war zone, perhaps. And that's about the way many severely obese people view surgery: not as something to welcome, but after a certain point, as maybe their best remaining hope for relief from excruciating back and leg pain, sleeplessness, labored breathing, heart failure and uncontrolled diabetes.

> *Although it can be defeated by an uncooperative patient, anti-obesity surgery offers the motivated individual a clean break from past behavior patterns and a powerful tool to achieve consumption of less calories and, therefore, permanent weight loss.*

SURGERY OVERVIEW

These days, the outlook for anti-obesity surgery is much improved from decades ago, when side effects such as liver failure, metabolic diseases and a toxic-shock-type infection of the bypassed small intestine were not infrequent. After experimenting with more than 30 variations over the years, most weight-loss surgeons have settled on a small number of techniques that have a known list of side effects (planned consequences) and complications (unplanned consequences that sometimes occur despite everyone's best efforts). Some of these new surgeries are minimally invasive. They use laparoscopic techniques to thread the surgical instruments into the stomach or intestines along with a camera that allows remote viewing. Therefore, the surgical wounds (often called "keyholes") are smaller and recovery from the operation is quicker. Whether this new method will represent a better way of performing these highly complex operations in the long run is still not clear. Studies are under way.

Weight-loss surgeons say that, in the end, whatever technique is used, surgery offers severely obese people their best chance for lasting weight loss.

"For the very overweight, surgery is the only approach that has proved to provide effective, safe, and durable weight control," write the authors of a recent scholarly review, summarizing more than 45 years of experience in the field since the first operations were performed.[1]

Long-term measures of obesity treatment are hard to come by. Groups that have been studied for more than several years following any form of treatment *other* than surgery are rare. Whether antiobesity surgery is the only successful long-term treatment for morbid obesity, therefore, is open to debate. But there is no denying that it is *among* the most successful treatments—for many morbidly obese people, perhaps, their last, best hope.

One of the best-known comparisons of surgical versus nonsurgical treatments is the Swedish Obese Subjects (SOS) study, which was started in 1987 and continues today. The researchers' goal is to match 2,000 people who receive surgical treatment for obesity with 2,000 people who do not, and to follow each pair for 10 years to see how they fare. By early 2000, researchers had enrolled 1,879 pairs in the study and reported the following results:

> *Weight-loss surgeons say that, in the end, whatever technique is used, surgery offers severely obese people their best chance for lasting weight loss.*

- After 2 years, surgical patients had achieved an average weight reduction of 28 kilograms (nearly 62 pounds), whereas nonsurgical patients had lost 0.5 kilograms (about 1 pound). After 8 years, the average weight loss in the surgical group was 20 kilograms (about 44 pounds), whereas nonsurgical patients had actually gained an average of 0.7 kilograms (about 1.5 pounds).

- After 2 years, the incidence of diabetes declined 32 times as much in the surgical patients as in the nonsurgical patients.

After 8 years, the decline was still five times as great in the surgical group.
- After 2 years, the reduction in hypertension (high blood pressure) was 2.6 times greater in the surgical than in the nonsurgical group. After eight years, however, the incidence of hypertension in the two groups was equal.
- It is "still too early to tell" whether the weight loss in either group will translate into overall lower mortality, i.e., longer life.[2]

Perhaps not surprisingly, in Sweden as in the United States, this study coincides with a period of rapidly increasing use of obesity surgery. (Unlike the United States, Sweden has a national system of health-care insurance and, therefore, keeps uniform statistics on all hospital cases in the country, making comprehensive comparisons such as the SOS study possible.) In the 9-year period between 1987 and 1996, Swedish surgeons performed nearly 7,200 obesity surgeries, with the annual number tripling during the study period. Slightly more than three-fourths of these surgeries were performed on women, at an average age of 39. Only 0.4 percent of the surgeries resulted in patient deaths, but by 1996, 14 percent of the surgeries being performed—nearly one in seven—were reoperations. "The operative mortality is low, but the incidence of a second obesity procedure is high," the researchers concluded.[3] It is also important to note that the SOS study is not a controlled trial—that is, the choice of whether or not to have surgery is not assigned by a coin toss, but by the patient and physician. Thus, it is not possible to truly match patients with a comparison group, as the motivations of the patients and controls are likely to differ, and this may affect how they do down the road.

Once again, we see that there is no magic bullet—or surgical sword, as the case may be—in the fight against obesity. However, surgery is one of the most powerful weapons doctors have. And most weight-management professionals turn to it without hesitation when circumstances warrant.

Who Should Have Surgery?

Surgery is recommended only for the severely obese who have not been able to lose weight in any other way, despite their efforts. That means it is a choice of last resort for people with BMIs of 40 or above, or people with BMIs of 35 or above along with serious associated medical conditions that are considered life-threatening, such as severe type 2 diabetes, sleep apnea, or heart disease. In practice, this often translates into men who are 100 pounds or more above their ideal body weight, or women who are 80 pounds or more above their ideal body weight. Given the sharp rise in the number of obese individuals over the past generation (as discussed in chapters 1 and 2), it is estimated that about 10 million people in the United States fall into this category.[4] This represents a doubling of the proportion of adults who are severely obese. Bariatric surgeons believe that many, if not most, of these people are potential candidates for obesity surgery. Paralleling the rapid increase seen in Sweden, the number of bariatric surgeries in the United States doubled from 20,000 in 1995 to about 40,000 in 2000.[5]

Currently, the American Society for Bariatric Surgery estimates its members are performing about 50,000 procedures a year—and indeed, its membership has grown by nearly 60 percent in the past two years, says executive director Georgeann Mallory.

Although the many problems with the earliest form of bariatric surgery, intestinal bypass, made many in the medical community leery of obesity surgery—and for good reason—the climate began to warm in 1991 when a National Institutes of Health Consensus Conference endorsed surgery as an acceptable form of treatment for many morbidly obese people. The NIH panel of experts concluded that there

> *Surgery is recommended only for the severely obese who have not been able to lose weight in any other way, despite their efforts. That means it is a choice of last resort for people with BMIs of 40 or above, or people with BMIs of 35 or above along with serious associated medical conditions that are considered life-threatening.*

are major drawbacks to all other forms of treatment for the severely obese. They found that people enrolled in Very Low Calorie Diets (VLCDs), who often can achieve a weight loss of more than 40 pounds in a few months under medical supervision, usually do not keep that weight off for a year. By the same token, proof of the long-term effectiveness of exercise and behavior modification was lacking, the panel said, and treatment with weight-reduction drugs has been "disappointing." The experts conceded that "limited success has been achieved by various techniques that include medically supervised dieting and intensive behavior modification.... The possibility should not be excluded that the highly motivated patient can achieve sustained weight reduction by a combination of supervised low-calorie diets and prolonged, intensive behavior modification therapy."[6]

With that rather doleful review of the alternatives, the panel concluded that surgical treatment for severe obesity "can induce substantial weight loss," and that, in turn, can produce improvement in associated disease conditions. Therefore, the panel concluded that obesity surgery makes sense for patients who are "well informed and motivated," who are able to participate in their own treatment and stay involved in the long-term follow-up that is required, and who "strongly desire substantial weight loss, because obesity severely impairs the quality of their lives."

> *The panel concluded that obesity surgery makes sense for patients who are "well informed and motivated," who are able to participate in their own treatment and stay involved in the long-term follow-up that is required, and who "strongly desire substantial weight loss, because obesity severely impairs the quality of their lives."*

Today, there is widespread agreement about how candidates for surgery should be evaluated and screened. Most surgeons will look for evidence that patients have tried, and failed, to lose weight in a *medically supervised program* of behavior modification and dietary counseling. Go-it-alone attempts don't count. If patients have not had this experience, they will often be referred to a medically based weight-management program first.

This is because obesity surgery is a serious operation. Although only a minority of seriously obese people are able to achieve sustained weight loss through dietary programs alone, the fact that some can do so makes it worth the attempt. Surgery is a treatment of last resort that is justified by the severity of the condition it attempts to cure. As the American Society for Bariatric Surgery states in a rather careful choice of words: "The option of surgical treatment is a rational one supported by the time-honored principle that diseases that harm call for therapeutic intervention that is less harmful than the disease being treated."[7]

Also important is evaluation by a psychiatrist or psychologist to exclude people who are alcoholic, substance abusers, or suffering from a major psychiatric illness. Prospective candidates must agree to change their diets and their eating behavior for the rest of their lives. In a real sense, there is no going back. Although procedures can, in theory, be reversed, second operations are even more risky than the first. At the most basic level, surgeons and psychologists must have reasonable confidence that surgical candidates will take a multivitamin supplement every day for the rest of their lives. The American Society for Bariatric Surgery acknowledges, however, that psychological evaluation is of "limited value" in separating winners from losers prior to surgery.[8]

A special warning must be offered to women of childbearing age. About four out of five obesity-surgery patients—80 percent—fall into this category. They must agree to take strict birth-control measures to ensure they do not become pregnant within two years following the surgery. Most weight loss occurs within 18 to 24 months after surgery. A woman who becomes pregnant during this period will not ingest enough nutrition to support her own needs and those of a developing fetus. Ironically, this is just when women who were previously infertile because of extreme obesity may regain the ability to conceive. With appropriate medical care following the two-year timetable, some women have been able to become pregnant and give birth to healthy babies.[9]

And finally, though some surgeons disagree, many will not operate on people who are younger than 16 or older than 65. "We've operated on several patients in college and they do just fine," says Dr. Thomas Magnuson, chief of general surgery at the Johns Hopkins Bayview Medical Center in Baltimore, who draws the line at age 18. "Operating on adolescents, however, is controversial because they may not have achieved their full growth potential yet. Therefore, if you do an operation that inhibits their ability to get calories, people argue that long-term, that could be detrimental to the patient."

What Are the Surgical Options?

The first weight-reduction surgeries were performed in the 1950s. They involved creating new pathways for food after it left the stomach, bypassing most of the small intestine. Known as "malabsorptive" procedures, the early intestinal bypasses connected the beginning and end segments of the small intestine together, bypassing the segment in between, which excludes more than 18 feet of its 20-foot length. This drastically reduced the number of calories the body could absorb from meals, as much of the body's digestion of nutrients and calories occurs in the small intestine. The early intestinal bypasses had an unacceptably high rate of deaths due to liver failure and kidney failure, along with long-term complications such as diarrhea, arthritis, hepatitis, cirrhosis, chronic kidney disease, hair loss, anemia, osteoporosis, and osteomalacia (a painful condition of softening and weakening bones).[10]

Beginning in the 1960s, surgeons began refining a less drastic but still effective type of operation, the gastric bypass, which channeled food into the small intestine after traveling through only a small portion of the stomach. Dr. Ed-

> *The early intestinal bypasses had an unacceptably high rate of deaths due to liver failure and kidney failure, along with long-term complications such as diarrhea, arthritis, hepatitis, cirrhosis, chronic kidney disease, hair loss, anemia, osteoporosis, and osteomalacia (a painful condition of softening and weakening bones).*

ward Mason, professor emeritus of surgery at the University of Iowa, began using gastric bypass for the treatment of obesity in 1966, following a series of successful experiments with dogs. "All we did was to take the operation that had been in use for 50 years for treatment of peptic ulcer, and which was actually being abandoned because of its side effects, and use the most important side effect, the inability to maintain body weight, for the treatment of severe obesity," he says.

Dr. Mason went on to develop the vertical banded gastroplasty (VBG), which restricts food intake by coupling the use of a restrictive band (a type of plastic belt) with a vertical line of surgical staples to create a small pouch in the stomach (see figure 5.1). There is a small opening in the bottom of the pouch—about one-quarter-inch wide—leading to the lower stomach and the small intestine. This pouch, then, becomes the intake valve for food coming "down the hatch" from the esophagus. And it drastically limits the flow. The ordinary stomach can hold 3 pints of food at a time—about 48 ounces' worth. A stomach pouch that has been created by a bariatric surgeon can hold only about an ounce of food immediately following surgery—"about the size of a shot glass," says one surgeon. Over time, it might stretch to no more than 2 or 3 ounces' worth. This has the effect of drastically reducing the amount of food that the patient can eat at any given time. In effect, he *must* eat slowly and chew thoroughly, or gagging, nausea, and vomiting will ensue. Patients literally take their food a teaspoon at a time.

On the plus side, many of those who have undergone gastric restriction say they experience feelings of fullness, or satiety, from quantities of food they would have laughed at before their surgery.

> These days, the obesity operation performed most often in the United States is actually a hybrid of the earlier intestinal bypass and the gastric restriction surgeries.

These days, the obesity operation performed most often in the United States is actually a hybrid of the earlier intestinal bypass and the gastric restriction surgeries. It is called the "Roux-en-Y" gastric bypass, after the Y-shaped connection formed during the rerouting of the stomach and the intestines (see figure 5.2).

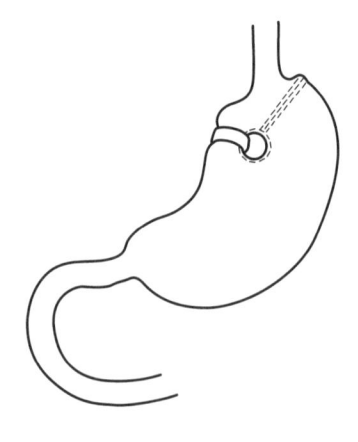

Figure 5.1—*Vertical Banded Gastroplasty*

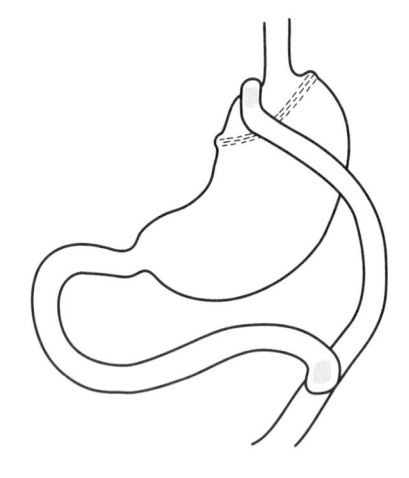

Figure 5.2—*Roux-en-Y Gastric Bypass*

In the Roux-en-Y, a small pouch is created in the stomach with a line of surgical staples. A segment of the small intestine is then attached to the small pouch through a *stoma,* or an opening in the side of the stomach. This segment is referred to as the *Roux-en-Y limb*. This creates a new GI tract. Food comes from the esophagus into the stomach pouch; it then leaves the stomach through the stoma and proceeds through the Roux-en-Y limb of the small intestine, bypassing the great bulk of the stomach as well as approximately the first 2 feet of the small intestine, consisting of the duodenum and part of the jejunum. Patients will tend to lose weight both because they physically cannot eat as much food at any one time, *and* because some of the caloric value of the food they eat will be lost as it is rerouted past the upper coils of the small intestine where it would ordinarily be absorbed into the bloodstream. Because most of the iron and calcium from food is absorbed in the duodenum, anemia, vitamin-B_{12} deficiency, and osteoporosis are all potential risks of the Roux-en-Y, especially for women who are still menstruating. Patients must take multivitamins faithfully for the rest of their lives; they may also be required to take iron and calcium supplements.[11] Some surgeons, including Dr. Mason, worry that there may be long-term nutritional and metabolic complications associated with the Roux-en-Y that will not become apparent until more decades have passed. But most practitioners believe that nutritional supplements will protect the health of patients.

Next in popularity in the United States is the vertical banded gastroplasty (VBG), described earlier. Used least of all, but sometimes required for "superobese" patients, is the *biliopancreatic diversion (BPD)*. Something of a throwback to the early days of intestinal bypass, this involves the removal of part of the stomach and the bypass of most of the small intestine. This surgery can achieve the greatest amount of weight loss that is currently attainable, but careful lifelong management of the patient is required to avoid serious nutritional and metabolic complications, including protein malnutrition and ulcers. Although patients can eat almost normally, there are unpleasant side effects, including loose and foul-smelling stools and unpleasant body odor. The procedure's inventor, Dr. Nicola Scopinaro of Genoa, Italy, has reported that at an 18-year follow-up, his patients had lost an average of 72 percent of excess weight.[12]

Finally, just beginning to be used in the United States (following FDA approval) is what has become the surgery of choice in much of Europe—the *laparoscopically adjustable gastric band*, which will be discussed later in this chapter.

What Are the Risks and Side Effects of Surgery?

There are many complications and side effects of obesity surgery, but the one that many patients will want to consider first and last, understandably, is death. Although unusual, it does happen. A panel of obesity experts convened by the National Institutes of Health reviewed all the pertinent literature on the subject and concluded, not surprisingly, that patient mortality differs markedly according to the types of patients in question. (Surgeons sometimes refer to the variation in types of patients as "patient selection"; it is one of many crucial variables that make comparing one surgeon's success

> *A panel of obesity experts convened by the National Institutes of Health reviewed all the pertinent literature on the subject and concluded, not surprisingly, that patient mortality differs markedly according to the types of patients in question.*

What a Surgery Patient Should Look For

The prestigious American College of Surgeons, at the request of the American Society of Bariatric Surgery, recently developed a list of recommended standards for surgeons and facilities performing obesity operations. The purpose of these guidelines, which were published in 2000, is to promote excellence in surgical care and patient safety.

Patients who are considering bariatric surgery would be well advised to compare the surgeons or hospitals they are considering with these guidelines. The full article may be consulted on the Internet at www.facs.org/fellows_info/statements/st-34.html. Following is a summary:

- **Surgeons** should be certified by the American Board of Surgery, or in the process of achieving such certification, and should have experience and technical skills in bariatric surgery. They should be committed to following patients long-term after surgery with an interdisciplinary team.

- **Bariatric-surgery management team** should include, in addition to the surgeon, skilled nurses, nutritionists, anesthesiologists with special training and experience and, as needed, endocrinologists, psychiatrists, cardiologists, pulmonologists (specialists in lung diseases), psychiatrists or psychologists, and specialists in physical rehabilitation.

- **Operating room and other facilities** should include special radiology equipment that may be required for preoperative examination of massively obese patients, as well as tables and other equipment that can accommodate patients weighing up to 750 pounds. These patients may also require special beds, chairs, commodes, and wheelchairs.

- **Recovery room staff** should include specialists in caring for patients with special ventilator and respirator needs.

- **Long-term care** following surgery should include physical rehabilitation, psychiatric counseling, nutritional counseling, and patient-support-group meetings.

In addition to these general guidelines from the American College of Surgeons, patients who are contemplating bariatric surgery should follow the same commonsense rules as anyone else selecting a surgeon for a high-risk procedure. You have a right to know how many operations like yours the surgeon you are considering has performed. *The more, the better.* Many studies show that doing a high volume of the same operation, over and over, breeds excellence, not only in a surgeon, but in the entire surgical team that must function as a well-rehearsed unit. In general, what is the surgeon's track record? How many patients fitting your profile died (if any), and how did they die? How many patients required reoperation because of complications? How many patients have successfully kept off weight 5 years after surgery? Ask to speak with other patients who have been treated by this surgeon. Would they do it again? You should ask for at least as many references as you would in choosing a contractor to build a deck on your house.

Don't be bashful. Remember, this is your body, and you are about to change it permanently. Good surgeons understand this and will give you as much information as you need to make an informed decision. The membership list of the American Society for Bariatric Surgery is available online at www.asbs.org/html/member.html.

rate to another surgeon's so difficult.) In general, the panel said, younger patients, with a BMI of less than 50 and no associated diseases, have mortality rates of less than 1 percent, whereas "massively obese" patients, with a BMI of 60 or above and associated medical conditions such as diabetes, hypertension, and heart and lung failure, may have mortality rates of 2 to 4 percent.[13]

Dr. Magnuson advises his patients that obesity surgery may have a 1 to 2 percent mortality rate. That includes death from all causes within 30 days of the operation. Though he has never lost a patient under 40 within 30 days of surgery, he says older patients and massively obese patients are more risky. "If you're operating on 20-year-olds who weigh 250 pounds, surgical mortality is real low," he says. "If you take all comers and you're operating on people who are 600 pounds, then your mortality is pretty high. But the mortality of not doing anything is probably higher. The 1-year mortality of a 600-pound patient with sleep apnea, congestive heart failure, and diabetes has got to be at least 15 percent. When you're 600 pounds and you can't move, you're going to die. So even though the operative mortality is also high, it's always a risk-benefit kind of thing."

Potential causes of operative mortality are the same as for other major types of abdominal surgery, including infection following leakage from the stomach into the abdominal cavity and the formation of blood clots leading to stroke or pulmonary embolism. Major complications can also include an adverse reaction to anesthesia (as in any surgery), injury to organs such as the esophagus or spleen, bowel obstruction due to adhesions or scarring, and wound infection.

Other risks, while perhaps not as dramatic, are nevertheless unpleasant.

Gallstones. A major complication of rapid weight loss (more than 1 pound a week) is the formation of gallstones. These painful accumulations of cholesterol, bile pigments, and calcium salts will form in up to one-third of patients undergoing obesity surgery. This can be avoided either by the removal of the gallbladder at the time of surgery (assuming one remains) or by the consumption of bile salt supplements for 6 months following surgery.

Conditions requiring reoperation. As many as 10 to 20 percent of all patients may require reoperation for problems such as leakage from the stomach or intestines; abdominal hernias; erosion and tearing of the staple line used to create the stomach pouch; or stomach outlets that stretch too far.[14]

One study that followed more than 600 gastric-bypass patients for 14 years found the complications listed in table 6.

Table 6. Gastric Bypass Surgery Complications: 14-Year Follow-Up

Complication	Patients Affected
Vitamin B_{12} deficiency	39.9%
Readmission to hospital (all reasons)	38.2%
Incisional hernia	23.9%
Depression	23.7%
Staple-line failure	15.0%
Gastritis (inflamed stomach lining)	13.2%
Cholecystitis (inflamed gallbladder)	11.4%
Anastomatic problems (site of bypass)	9.8%
Dehydration, malnutrition	5.8%
Dilated pouch	3.2%

Source: National Heart, Lung, and Blood Institute, "Clinical Guidelines on the Identification, Evaluation, and Treatment of Overweight and Obesity in Adults," in *Obesity Research* 6, supplement 2 (September 1998).

The list of complications from the vertical banded gastroplasty is shorter. Most important, perhaps, because it does not depend on bypassing any part of the small intestine, patients do not need to worry about the malabsorptive problems of anemia, osteoporosis, and the like.[15] Nor do they suffer from the "dumping syndrome" leading to weakness, sweating, and diarrhea after eating sweets. However, complications can include leaking, stenosis (partial obstruction of the opening in the pouch leading to vomiting), ulcer, hernia, infection of the wound, and erosion of the band around the stomach—another long-term problem whose effects, by definition, have not been studied for the decades that many patients expect to live.

The list of side effects (expected consequences) is no less daunting, according to a compilation of many published results of gastric bypass surgery (see table 7).

What Are the Benefits of Surgery?

First and foremost, surgery gets results. For all the trouble it may cause, it works. Various studies have found that a majority of patients

Table 7. Gastric Bypass Surgery Side Effects

Side Effects	Patients Affected
"Dumping syndrome"	70%
Dairy intolerance	50%
Constipation	40%
Headache	40%
Hair loss	33%
Depression	15%

Source: J. G. Kral, "Surgical Treatment of Obesity," in *Handbook of Obesity*, ed. G. A. Bray, C. Bouchard, and W. P. T. James (New York: Dekker, 1998).

(not all) lose up to half their excess weight with the VBG and up to two-thirds of their excess weight with the gastric bypass. Over time, patients gain some of their weight back. One of the best-known long-term studies, the "Greenville series" of more than 600 gastric-bypass patients at East Carolina University, found that the loss of excess weight averaged 50 percent at 14 years following surgery. Because it has some of the malabsorptive features involved in intestinal bypass, gastric bypass will lead, on average, to 10 to 15 percent more weight reduction than VBG. For the same reason, in turn, BPD (biliopancreatic diversion) produces even more substantial weight losses than gastric bypass, though with more complications and side effects, as described earlier.

> Various studies have found that a majority of patients (not all) lose up to half their excess weight with the VBG and up to two-thirds of their excess weight with the gastric bypass. Over time, patients gain some of their weight back.

Overall, obesity-surgery patients lose 25 to 40 percent of their pre-operation weight, says Dr. John Kral of the State University of New York at Brooklyn.[16] Obesity surgery, by substantially reducing the percentage of overweight, can lead, therefore, to sharp improvements in a broad range of medical conditions. Table 8 summarizes some of these benefits, based on data from more than 1,000 patients.

A long-term study in North Carolina, the Greenville series mentioned above, found that 83 percent of patients with type 2 diabetes who underwent gastric bypass were cured at 14 years postsurgery. "To our knowledge, gastric bypass is the only therapy ever reported to reduce the mortality from type 2 diabetes mellitus," write Drs. R. J. Albrecht and W. J. Pories.[17]

The Course of Treatment After Surgery

Postsurgical patients meet at regular intervals with their surgeon to monitor their progress. They are also encouraged to participate in patient-support groups. Strict compliance with their nutritional

Table 8. Effects of Surgery on Serious Diseases Associated with Obesity

Disease	Prevalence	"Cured"[a]	Improved[b]
Hypertension	30–60%	60–65%	90%
Diabetes	15–20%	90–95%	100%
Dyslipidemia	15–25%	70%	85%
Asthma	10–15%	> 95%	100%
Heart failure	10%	60%	90%
Sleep apnea	2–5%	100%	100%

Source: Adapted from J. G. Kral, "Surgical Treatment of Obesity," in *Treatment of the Seriously Obese Patient*, ed. T. A. Wadden and T. B. VanItallie (New York: Guilford, 1992).

Notes: a. Absence of symptoms with no further need for medication.
b. Reduced medication dosage.

program is crucial. Changing dietary habits and eating behavior is key to their success or failure. *Even weight-loss surgery can be defeated if patients fail to get with the program.*

Patients learn quickly that eating too fast produces nausea and vomiting. But they must also change the type of foods they eat. After the gastric bypass, eating sweet, high-calorie junk foods—such as ice cream, cookies, cheese, and cake—can trigger the "dumping syndrome," as these foods quickly reach a segment of the small intestine that does not ordinarily receive calorie-laden foods in such quantity. Patients sweat, flush, have heart palpitations, feel nauseated, and suffer from diarrhea. High-calorie drinks can also trigger these symptoms, especially alcohol and soda.

Patients with a VBG (gastric banding) are not susceptible to the dumping syndrome, and for that reason some experts believe a subset of these patients has a tendency to become "sweet-eaters." They may even consume their excess calories by drinking them in the form of soft drinks or other sweet beverages. No matter what type of surgery has been done, patients can defeat it over time by eating or nibbling constantly on high-fat or high-carbohydrate foods.[18]

"People that fail the surgery tend to fail because they go back to snacking and grazing behavior," says Dr. Charles Callery, a bariatric surgeon with a private practice in the San Diego area.[19] However, right off the bat, and for the first 6 months or so after surgery, "people do fine," he says. "Then it's all over the map."

In Dr. Callery's practice, patients are followed intensively after surgery. Early on, they meet three times a month with support groups, then two times a month. The surgeon sees them at 1 week, 2 weeks, 3 months, 6 months, 9 months, 18 months, and 2 years after surgery—by which time, experience says they will have achieved virtually all of their weight loss. They are also counseled by a psychologist and a dietitian.

> *No matter what type of surgery has been done, patients can defeat it over time by eating or nibbling constantly on high-fat or high-carbohydrate foods.*

On the average, Dr. Callery says his Roux-en-Y patients will have lost about three-fourths of their excess weight (78 percent) at 2 years, which is in line with published results elsewhere. After reaching their lowest post-operative weight, they tend to gain some weight back, leveling off at about two-thirds excess weight loss at 4 years following surgery. But individual results vary greatly.[20] He finds that a lucky minority of his patients—perhaps 20 percent—experience a kind of transformation in their relationship to food. "Surgery does something physiologically or psychologically that dramatically changes the patient's desire for and appreciation of food. . . . I have some patients that say, 'I just eat whatever I like; it's like I was never fat before.'"

On the other extreme are about 20 percent of those who cannot modify their eating habits or who for some reason do not benefit as much from the surgery. They may succeed in shedding only about one-quarter of their excess weight. "You've got some patients who are still struggling, just like they were when they came in. They don't lose very much weight, and they don't know what the problem is."

The majority of people—maybe 60 percent—will experience success, but at the price of continued effort. "You've got that middle group of patients who do have to think about what they're eating, and they do have to consciously push the plate away when they start to feel full."

Dr. Magnuson, like Dr. Callery, notes that most patients are *compliant*—the medical term for doing what their doctor tells them to do. "Even though diets didn't work in the past, for some reason they are able to handle the operation, and they are able to modify their eating habits. Whether that's some kind of psychological thing, in that they've

---

Ten Rules for Success Following Bariatric Surgery

Dietitians at the Johns Hopkins Weight Management Center who work with gastric-bypass patients offer the following rules for a successful outcome to this complicated surgery:

1. Eat six small meals each day. After the initial adaptation period, each meal should be approximately 3 to 4 ounces of food, including protein, starch, and vegetable or fruit.
2. Eat protein foods (lean meats, lowfat cheese and yogurt, eggs and soy products) first, followed by vegetables or fruits and then starches and grains.
3. Stop eating as soon as you feel full or when you have finished the allotted amount of food (3 to 4 ounces). Do not eat more than the amount your stomach is comfortable handling.
4. Do not drink while you are eating. Taking liquids while you are eating solid food may cause the solid foods to empty too quickly from the stomach outlet.

invested in a major operation, or whether the operation somehow resets some kind of sensor in their brain and makes it better for them, is unclear." The real struggles with compliance are not in losing weight, but in eating properly, taking multivitamins and other supplements, and avoiding metabolic complications from nutritional imbalance, he says.

Dr. John Kral of the State University of New York at Brooklyn, reviewing the long-term Greenville study of gastric bypass, says there is a failure rate of about 20 percent, where failure is defined as not being able to keep off enough excess weight to avoid the comorbidities (diabetes, sleep apnea, and the like) that made surgery necessary in the first place.[21] He observes that surgeries can fail for several major reasons: "aggressive overeating," leading to stretching of the

---

5. Avoid high-calorie and high-fat foods such as ice cream, baked goods, cheeses, sweetened sodas, and alcohol. They may deter weight loss or cause regaining of weight.
6. Eat foods that provide essential nutrients, such as fresh vegetables, fruit, lean meat, and cereals. Avoid fruit juices and drinks, which are relatively high-calorie and pass quickly through the pouch, causing "dumping syndrome."
7. Avoid fibrous foods such as asparagus and celery, which can block the stomach outlet. Other foods that may be difficult to digest include red meats, white bread, and pasta.
8. Drink six to eight glasses of water per day. Tea and coffee are also permitted, but without cream or sugar.
9. Begin exercising with your physician's approval. Swimming and walking are low-impact activities that can get you back into the swing of moving your body.
10. Subject to your physician's approval, take a multivitamin with minerals every day.

stomach pouch, breakdown of the staple lines, or erosion of the gastric band; "maladaptive eating," in which patients seek out soft, rich foods that pass through the small outlet; and "gradual adaptation" of the lining of the small intestine, which in turn diminishes the "dumping syndrome" that requires bypass patients to avoid ice cream and other sweets.[22]

What Can Surgery Patients Eat?

In the first week or two after surgery, the restrictions will sound familiar for anyone who has had an operation. Patients must stick to a largely liquid diet—broth, tea, coffee, flat diet soda (the bubbles that make the fizz can cause trouble), liquid gelatin, unsweetened fruit juices. In weeks 2 through 6, patients can graduate to lowfat, low-sugar foods such as skim milk, sugar-free or low-cal gelatins and custards, breads and crackers, rice and pasta, cereals, lowfat yogurt and cottage cheese, eggs, well-cooked vegetables, soft fruits, and meats such as pâté, shrimp, and fish. Later, some specialists recommend protein supplements mixed with juice or soup; soy-meat supplements; and virtually any kind of meat, well cooked and cut into very small pieces (see www.thinnertimes.com for further recommendations). "Many [patients] report the ability to eat half a hamburger, some French fries and a small glass of diet soft drink after about 6 months," report Albrecht and Pories.[23]

> Gastric-bypass patients should avoid those awfully tempting, high-calorie goodies such as ice cream, chocolate, regular cheese, and cookies, lest they trigger the "dumping syndrome," complete with nausea, sweating, and diarrhea.

No-No's

Gastric-bypass patients should avoid those awfully tempting, high-calorie goodies such as ice cream, chocolate, regular cheese, and cookies, lest they trigger the "dumping syndrome," complete with nausea, sweating, and diarrhea. Patients must avoid alcohol and sweetened sodas. And finally, they can actually clog their pouches if they eat meat that is not well cooked, certain fruit skins, bread made with refined flour, and wide noodles, Johns Hopkins advises its patients.

Paying for the Operation

Bariatric surgeries typically cost about $15,000 to $20,000, including both surgeons' and hospital fees. Dr. Magnuson estimates that 80 to 90 percent of patients who are referred for surgery by another doctor are able to get coverage from their health-insurance company. Sometimes appeal is necessary, but approval usually follows. Two North Carolina surgeons note that insurance refusals are "uncommon" following the classification of severe obesity with complicating conditions as a disease in the Americans with Disabilities Act.[24]

WHAT'S NEW: LAPAROSCOPICALLY ADJUSTABLE GASTRIC BANDS

In much of the world, one of the most common obesity surgeries is a laparoscopic implant procedure that was only approved in this country by the Food and Drug Administration in June 2001. Many surgeons around the country are waiting to see whether its track record improves and how it is received by the public. There seems to be little doubt that this new approach could become the obesity surgery of choice in the United States, as well, if it can overcome a somewhat mixed record in clinical trials, which saw a 25-percent reoperation rate due to unpleasant side effects and a general failure to work in some cases.

In this procedure, surgeons wrap a plastic band around the stomach, called the *Laparoscopically adjustable gastric band*, or LAP-band (see figure 5.3). The band is tightened, as in the gastric restriction surgeries. Because the stomach is smaller, patients feel fuller more quickly when they eat and cannot eat as much as they ordinarily do. The LAP-band system has several features that are appealing to many patients.

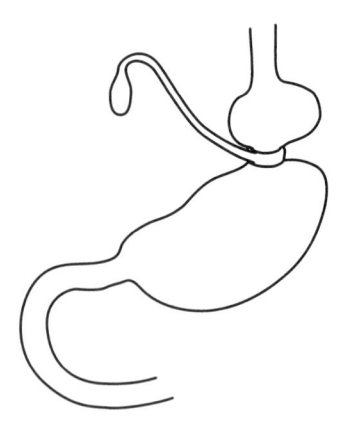

Figure 5.3—*The Laparoscopically Adjustable Gastric Band*

It is implanted *laparoscopically*. Instead of a large surgical wound allowing the surgeon to clearly see the entire field of operation, several small keyhole incisions are made, and the operation is done at the end of a long, flexible tube while the surgeon follows the operation's progress on a TV monitor. Surgeons differ on whether laparoscopic surgery produces a better outcome in an operation this complex. But assuming all goes well, the surgical wounds heal more quickly. (In the clinical trials, about 5 percent of the implantations were done in "open" surgery because of problems the surgeon encountered laparoscopically.)

The surgery is *modifiable*. The LAP-band itself is connected to a small reservoir, implanted beneath the patient's skin. Fluid flows from the reservoir into the band, similar to an inner tube that can be inflated or deflated with air. In this case, the surgeon injects a saline solution into the LAP-band's reservoir with a fine needle. When solution is added, the LAP-band swells and restricts the stomach more tightly. When solution is withdrawn, the LAP-band relaxes, the stomach can expand, and the patient can eat more. This may be particularly useful, for instance, to women who become pregnant and therefore need more nutrition.

The surgery is *reversible*. Although it is not anyone's goal to bring it back out, the LAP-band can be removed if side effects and complications make that desirable. It is, in a sense, a purely mechanical device. Although the stomach may be sutured (stitched), no stomach tissue is stapled, nor are any of the intestines cut and bypassed. Sometimes the LAP-band can be removed laparoscopically, but sometimes open surgery is required.

In approving the device, the FDA set down a series of conditions for the manufacturer, BioEnterics Corporation of Carpinteria, California:

- It is indicated for use only in patients who are severely obese (BMI of 40 or above, or BMI of 35 or above with serious comorbidities).
- Patients must have tried and failed "more conservative" weight-loss programs, including diet, exercise, and behavior modification.
- Patients must commit themselves to make "significant changes in their eating habits for the rest of their lives."[25]

The LAP-band system has several features that are appealing to many patients: It is implanted laparoscopically, the surgery is modifiable, and the surgery is reversible.

The FDA based its approval on company-sponsored clinical trials involving 299 patients, ages 18 to 55, at eight sites. The patients were required to follow a strict diet and to exercise daily following the operation. At the beginning of the 3-year trial, the patients' mean (average) weight was 293 pounds. They were overweight by an average of 156 pounds, with a BMI of more than 47. After 3 years of wearing the LAP-band, their average weight decreased to 241 pounds, their overweight to about 98 pounds, and their BMI to less than 39. There were, however, some exceptions. Ten percent of the patients lost 75 percent of their excess weight, at the one extreme, whereas 5 percent did not lose any weight, and 2 percent actually gained weight, at the other extreme.

However, there were a number of what the FDA termed "adverse events," including the following:

- Nausea and vomiting (51 percent)
- Gastroesophageal reflux, or heartburn (34 percent)

- Abdominal pain (27 percent)
- Slippage of the band, leading to expansion of the stomach pouch (24 percent)
- Obstruction of the stoma, or stomach outlet (14 percent)
- Constipation (9 percent)
- Swallowing difficulties (9 percent)
- Pain at the port site where the reservoir is refilled (9 percent)

In 75 cases, or one-quarter of all patients, the system was removed entirely, mostly because of the negative side effects. Nine percent of the patients needed a reoperation to correct a problem.[26]

By the summer of 2002, the LAP-band should be available at about 200 sites in the United States, said Don Mills, communications manager for BioEnterics. He said the company will only sell the band to skilled laparoscopic surgeons who go through a special training program from BioEnterics. Worldwide, he said, about 70,000 of the LAP-bands had been implanted prior to U.S. approval.

HOW ABOUT PLASTIC SURGERY?

Bariatric surgery is a serious, life-altering procedure. But many Americans believe there is a quicker, easier way to get rid of fat: Just zap it with liposuction. And indeed, there may be some truth to that when it comes to those irritating bumps and bulges that won't go away, no matter how much straining or sweating we do, whether they're the "saddlebags" on women's thighs or the "love handles" on men's flanks.

In 2000, about 354,000 Americans had themselves scooped and sculpted in a liposuction procedure, according to the American Society of Plastic Surgeons.[27] An additional 62,700 had an abdominoplasty (tummy tuck), and 105,000 had breast reductions (including both men and women).

But both bariatric surgeons and plastic surgeons agree: Though there is a place for plastic surgery, it should not be confused with weight control.

The American Society for Bariatric Surgery states clearly that surgical treatment for morbid obesity is a medical necessity, not a cosmetic procedure; the professional societies for plastic and dermatologic surgery, on their part, freely acknowledge that liposuction should not be viewed as a means of weight control. "Tumescent liposuction [the leading technique, which involves injecting local anesthetic and large volumes of fluid into fatty areas before scooping them out with a vacuum wand] is not generally intended for weight loss but rather is a contouring procedure," says a statement from the American Society for Dermatologic Surgery. "It is best utilized in a program of exercise and optimal weight maintenance."[28]

In 2000, about 354,000 Americans had themselves scooped and sculpted in a liposuction procedure, according to the American Society of Plastic Surgeons. An additional 62,700 had an abdominoplasty (tummy tuck), and 105,000 had breast reductions (including both men and women).

The American Society for Plastic Surgery (ASPS) says that the best candidates for liposuction are "normal-weight people with firm, elastic skin who have pockets of excess fat in certain areas." The ASPS goes on to say, "Although no type of liposuction is a substitute for dieting and exercise, liposuction can remove stubborn areas of fat that don't respond to traditional weight-loss methods."[29]

Though liposuction, then, is available to those people who are only slightly overweight, or lumpy in the wrong places, it also has an important role to play for people who are recovering from traditional bariatric surgery.

When morbidly obese people lose 100 or more pounds, they can sometimes be left with massive, loose folds of skin, or large, droopy abdomens. In some cases these are merely cosmetic blemishes; in other cases, they can be challenges to personal hygiene or impediments to resuming a normal sex life.

Dr. Robert Jackson of Marion, Indiana, frequently performs liposuctions and abdominoplasties (tummy tucks) for people who have lost large amounts of weight following bariatric surgery. The president-elect of the American Academy of Cosmetic Surgery, Dr. Jackson operates on women who have lost up to 175 pounds. In one recent case involving a patient who shed 160 pounds following gastric bypass, he was able to suck out localized deposits of fat, remove excess folds of skin and fat that hung from the lower abdomen, and tighten the rectus muscles running up and down the abdomen. "In her case now, she has a flat abdomen," he said. "She could not get that with bariatric surgery alone. She could lose the weight, but she still had the extra skin."

Though there are no data on how many bariatric surgery patients need subsequent cosmetic surgery, the cases are not infrequent. Much depends on how extreme the weight loss was, how old the person was at the time of the weight loss, and how much elasticity was left in the skin. Many people will also want to know what to do about stretch marks. "There's not a lot you can do," says Dr. Jackson. "We've had some success with microderm abrasion, some laser therapy, also using retin-A and glycolic acid. We can't get rid of them totally. We can usually fade them a little bit. A lot of times when we do the removal of the skin and the tummy tucks, by tightening the skin, the stretch marks are still there but they don't show quite as bad."

> *Though there are no data on how many bariatric surgery patients need subsequent cosmetic surgery, the cases are not infrequent.*

As for Dr. Jackson, there is no denying that he is one doctor who takes his own medicine: In 1993, he had 6 to 7 pounds removed from his abdomen by liposuction.

WAYNE SMITH'S NEW LIFE

On October 7, 1999—his 60th birthday—Wayne Smith began a new life.

That's when he was implanted with the LAP-band gastric-restriction system, marking the end to a decades-long quest to find something that would help him lose weight. At 305 pounds, and with a BMI of 44, he had fortunately escaped many of the serious illnesses associated with severe obesity. He was healthy. But he was not satisfied.

His weight was interfering with his day-to-day life. He liked to drive street rods. But his stomach no longer fit behind the wheel. He liked to kayak. But he could not get out of his kayak once he got in. He liked to travel. But with a 64-inch waist, he couldn't pull the airline trays all the way down. When he wanted to put on his shoes, he had to grab a pant leg to pull his foot up to where he could reach it.

His weight became a problem for him when he was about 30, Smith says. He tried to diet his way out of it, and he tried to exercise his way out of it, but he always came up short.

"I tried taking up long-distance running, but that didn't work, because you hurt your ankles and your knees. And if you hit the ground wrong, you broke something. I went on Optifast three separate times, got all the way to goal weight, and put it all back on again in about two months."

Smith says one of those diets was in 1975, one was in 1980, one was in 1986. All of them were medically supervised. "In all cases, I went to goal," he says. "I got to 185 pounds, and then the minute you come off that very strict diet—400 calories a day—the body says, OK, time to pack it on. You eat 20 hamburgers at a time.

"I would go to work in the morning and hit McDonald's and get four or five of their big sandwiches and eat them before I got to work. And then coming home, particularly on those 39-cent days, I'd buy two dozen burgers, and kill them all before I got home. Then I could start eating like a bird again [at 300-plus pounds]."

In 1988, he started investigating obesity surgery. He says he talked to every bariatric surgeon in San Diego and four in Los Angeles. But what he heard scared him. As a former physics major, teacher, and software programmer, he felt there had to be a more straightforward way to do the procedure. "I put in my notes, 'Wouldn't it be a hell of a lot simpler if you took a rusty old radiator-hose clamp from a '57 Chevrolet and put that around your stomach?'" he says with a chuckle. "It would do identically the same all these guys were talking about, without the cutting and pasting."

A couple of years ago, he was browsing on the Internet when he stumbled across the LAP-band, which was then in clinical trials in the United States. He says he tried to enroll but was told he was too old. "Back I go to the Internet," he says. He found doctors doing laparoscopic surgery in Italy, Belgium, France, and Monterrey, Mexico. "I called [the Mexican doctor] up and said, 'How much?' He said, 'Six thousand, nine hundred dollars, plus the hospital fees.' I said, 'Book me.' I was on a plane the next day. I showed up in his office on a Wednesday afternoon. They did the blood work, they did the ECG, and I talked to the psychiatrist. . . . These guys were top-drawer all the way."

> Since the implantation, Smith has lost about 130 pounds. His weight loss is charted on his Web site, www.waynesmith.net.

After a 24-hour hospital stay, and three days longer in Monterrey, Smith returned to his San Diego home, sporting a LAP-band. Since then, he has been seen periodically by another Mexican doctor, in Tijuana, who lives about ten miles away from Smith. Since the implantation, Smith has lost about 130 pounds, he says. His weight loss is charted on his Web site, www.waynesmith.net, along with pictures of his surgical scars (minimal) and pictures of his steadily thinning self.

Smith, who left the computer business and is now happily employed as a school bus driver, says he has gone back and forth with fills and withdrawals from his LAP-band reservoir, trying to find the point that would maintain his weight at equilibrium. He thinks he has found it, as he has stayed within a 4-pound range for more than a year.

"Before the surgery I would eat anything and everything, and I ate it in large volume," he says cheerfully. "There was no restriction. I'd scarf down salads or roasts." Now he is into protein—chicken, fish, sardines—along with grits, rice, and couscous.

"But I can't eat near as much as I used to," he says. "I will admit to a strange feeling that I've had since I've gotten the band. Hunger. I actually do feel hungry. Before, I never had my mouth empty. I ate all the time, whether it was noon, breakfast, lunch, dinner, whatever. I ate."

With the LAP-band, he eats two meals a day. He takes very small bites—quarter-teaspoons, he says—and he chews them well. He almost always takes at least 20 minutes to eat a meal. He says he has not experienced any of the physical side effects such as nausea or vomiting.

With his new, lean frame, he can get up from the floor, unassisted. He can get out of his kayak without aid. He's got plenty of clearance when he slides behind the wheel of his street rod.

"I would have done this ages ago had I known it existed," he says emphatically. "Would I do it again? Yes. If the price were three times as much? Yes."

SUMMARY

For the severely obese who are at considerable risk of illness or death and who have not been able to lose weight by any other means, bariatric surgery is an answer of last resort. Doctors reserve this rather drastic procedure for patients who have a BMI of 40 and above, or 35 and above with serious comorbidities (illnesses associated with their obesity). The list of possible side effects from weight-reduction surgery, including death, is sobering. But the surgery has gotten safer as procedures have become more refined over the past 30 to 40 years. The latest techniques often make use of laparoscopic procedures, whereby doctors do not need to open the entire abdomen in order to create a gastric bypass or to place a plastic band around the stomach. Many surgeons and patients alike are waiting to see if the

> *For the severely obese who are at considerable risk of illness or death and who have not been able to lose weight by any other means, bariatric surgery is an answer of last resort.*

American experience with a laparoscopically adjustable stomach band will prove to be as successful as it seems to have been in Europe and elsewhere. In the meantime, when everything else has failed them, some patients find release in bariatric surgery from a lifetime imprisonment by their own weight.

CHAPTER 6

Complementary and Alternative Treatments

❦

NOT SURPRISINGLY, WEIGHT loss has spurred an enormous degree of interest in complementary and alternative treatments. These treatments, in large part, consist of nonmedical professionals taking matters into their own hands, largely because medical science has failed to help them. Diseases and conditions that are chronic, painful, and resistant to a straightforward cure are candidates for complementary and alternative solutions. The problem of overweight, whether it's characterized by 10 or 100 excess pounds in any individual case, falls into all of these categories.

It is *chronic*. As we have seen repeatedly in this book, losing weight is hard, especially when we are immersed in an extremely convenient, sedentary lifestyle, where few of us get the prescribed 30 minutes of vigorous exercise each day and most of us are surrounded by abundant helpings of fast food at every turn.

It is *painful*. Overweight and obesity are psychologically—and for many, physically—uncomfortable and distressing conditions.

And finally, as we have seen, there is no simple *cure* for overweight. Medical science has a clear answer for most people struggling with weight problems, which few are capable of implementing—eat less, exercise more. But beyond that maxim against which the body literally rebels, there is no remedy to request at the druggist's counter, at least not on a par with a dose of penicillin for pneumonia.

This means the chronic disorders of overweight and obesity—like those of back pain, cancer, and arthritis—have attracted a host of speculators and snake-oil salesmen as well as legitimate scientists, doctors, and other health professionals. Periodically, the Federal Trade Commission and the Food and Drug Administration have intervened to rein in the worst abuses of the times. But still, gimmicks and quick fixes abound, many wearing the halo of "natural herbs" or Asian "secret formulas." Alas, experience proves that "natural" products can be potent and, in some cases, just as damaging and deadly as pharmaceuticals—and their quality less assured because standards are rarely enforced by the federal government for products labeled as "dietary supplements" as opposed to drugs.

There are, however, alternative approaches—such as acupuncture—that have brought relief for some and which have their enthusiasts, even though they have not achieved mainstream acceptance. Perhaps they will someday; perhaps not.

> *There are, however, alternative approaches—such as acupuncture—that have brought relief for some and which have their enthusiasts, even though they have not achieved mainstream acceptance.*

The field of weight loss—for obvious reasons—has attracted more than its fair share of bogus claims. By this point in the book, it is probably clear what we think of any products or techniques that promise quick, painless, even "miracle" ways of bypassing the difficult life changes that are required for lasting weight loss. Yet just such promises abound in the tabloids, in many magazines, and on the Internet.

Yahoo!, the popular search engine, lists no fewer than 118 World Wide Web sites marketing weight-loss supplements, ranging from the scientifically well-founded to the flaky, and including many that combine a pinch of science with a large dollop of hype. Never has the phrase *caveat emptor*—"let the buyer beware"—been more appropriately applied. Here one can find a slimming chain to be worn around the waist, an electronic acupressure wristband, ancient Chinese seaweed soap that "melts the fat away," time-release aromatherapy to dull the appetite, body-contouring cream, fat-blocking dietary supplements, a hypnosis program, many herbal formulas, algae extracts, herbal teas, body wraps, fat-burners, fat-loss accelerators, and many more aids to slimming and trimming.[1]

The *New York Times* recently estimated that $6 billion a year is being spent by Americans on fraudulent diet products and that the rate has risen sharply since 1997, with the well-publicized withdrawal of the FDA-approved drugs fenfluramine and dexfenfluramine from the market.[2] The newspaper noted that "dieters have scrambled for a substitute that offers the same dramatic results with as little effort. In their search, they have turned quick-fix, over-the-counter weight-loss products from a tiny sliver of the diet industry into its fastest-growing segment."

An important perspective to keep in mind is that stated by Dr. Andrew Weil, one of the foremost interpreters (and proponents) of complementary and alternative therapies in the United States today. In words that virtually every medical professional would echo, he writes, "The important lesson dieters have to learn is that all calories count when you're trying to lose weight—and there is no magic pill that will allow you to lose weight without changing your eating habits. If you're trying to change your pants size, I can guarantee only one route to success: Eat less and exercise more."[3]

And again, "As for weight loss, my advice can be summed up in two words: Eat less."[4]

It is interesting to note that some of the hottest fads featured in magazines and on television really trade on these fundamentals—eat

> *The New York Times recently estimated that $6 billion a year is being spent by Americans on fraudulent diet products and that the rate has risen sharply since 1997, with the well-publicized withdrawal of the FDA-approved drugs fenfluramine and dexfenfluramine from the market.*

> **FTC's List of No-No's**
>
> Though almost every American who cares about health recognizes the crucial role of the Food and Drug Administration (FDA) in regulating drugs and medical devices, many people may not know of the important oversight responsibility of the Federal Trade Commission (FTC).
>
> With a mandate to enforce the nation's federal consumer-protection laws, the FTC has repeatedly brought charges against companies both large and small, well known and obscure, alleging that they engaged in deceptive advertising and made unsubstantiated claims about their weight-loss products and services. Most cases are settled with consent agreements, under which the companies agree to drop misleading ads and to stop making scientifically unproven claims.
>
> As fast as one case is settled, though, imitators seem to spring up. Therefore, alert readers may amuse themselves, as they flip through popular magazines or open e-mail marketing on the Web, by observing the eternal recurrence of certain themes that have attracted federal attention in the past.
>
> Just in the 1990s alone, the FTC brought more than 70 cases against the advertising claims of companies as well known as Weight Watchers and Jenny Craig, and as obscure as Bee Sweet and Body Wise International. It obtained consent agreements to drop misleading or unsubstantiated ads from firms marketing "Fat Burner" pills, acupressure ear clips, body wraps, chromium picolinate, skin patches, Super-Formulas, group-hypnosis seminars, MiracleTrim diet pills, cellulite-reducing creams, bee pollen, and many other overhyped goods and services. The FTC's targets also included some generally well-respected programs—such as Weight Watchers, Nutri/System,

less, exercise more. A recent magazine feature on trendy Hollywood diets included Ashtanga yoga, described as a "very physical form of yoga" that leads to "a leaner, more flexible body, stronger muscles and a clearer mind," and "cardio striptease," an hour-long aerobicize craze and Jenny Craig—whose advertising claims about their success rate, comparative superiority, and other features could not be substantiated to the FTC's satisfaction.[5]

In general, the settlements arrived at required these companies to be able to produce scientific data to prove any claims about weight loss they may make in the future; to base any claims about the long-term maintenance of weight loss on the actual experience of clients who had been followed for at least two years; to disclose all their fees to customers who inquired about them; and to correct certain other claims in their individual cases.[6]

As a guide to consumers, the FTC prepared the "Skinny on Dieting," a list of claims that should automatically make alarm bells go off:

- "Lose Weight While You Sleep." Claims of effortless weight loss are "bogus."
- "Lose Weight and Keep It Off for Good." Sure, but only if you make permanent changes in your eating and exercise patterns.
- "John Doe Lost 84 Pounds in 6 Weeks." Okay, but that may be totally irrelevant to you, even if true.
- "Lose All the Weight You Can for Just $99." Look out for hidden fees, such as the cost of mandatory meals you must buy from the program.
- "Lose 30 Pounds in Just 30 Days." Weight loss this fast can be dangerous, and difficult to keep off over the long haul.
- "Scientific Breakthrough . . . Medical Miracle." Rarely true. Hold on to your wallet.[7]

that encourages participants to shed clothes in order to show off their trimmer physiques.[8] Of course, any weight-loss success these programs have will depend on their ability to encourage more exercise on a regular basis, over a long period of time, in concert with a stable diet. The marketing may sound more beguiling, but the basics are familiar.

WHAT IS COMPLEMENTARY AND ALTERNATIVE MEDICINE?

Strictly speaking, *complementary* therapies are those that *supplement*, or enhance, conventional medical treatments. A therapy such as massage, which can be used together with and in support of conventional treatments such as chemotherapy or surgery, is a good example of a form of healing that is often classified as complementary medicine, but which is readily accepted by many mainstream physicians. Simply put, massage works to improve the sense of well-being, and to lessen pain and discomfort, in many people undergoing conventional treatments that will be the key to their cure.

However, some forms of massage could be classified as *alternative* (stand-alone) treatments—treatments such as "healing touch," which claim to bring about healing by manipulating bioenergy fields around the human body, for example. Alternative therapies such as this often rest on claims that are regarded as untested and literally incredible (unbelievable) by Western science.

At one time, not too many years ago, complementary and alternative medicine (CAM) was defined as those modes of treatment that were not taught in medical schools and not paid for by health-insurance companies. With increasing acceptance of at least some alternative methods—such as chiropractic and acupuncture—that old definition no longer suffices.

The National Center for Complementary and Alternative Medicine (NCCAM), a member body of the National Institutes of Health,

> At one time, complementary and alternative medicine was defined as those modes of treatment that were not taught in medical schools, and not paid for by health-insurance companies. With increasing acceptance of at least some alternative methods, that old definition no longer suffices.

states that complementary and alternative health-care and medical practices (CAM) fall into five main categories. Some types of treatment, such as acupuncture and herbal therapy, overlap these categories, which are therefore not mutually exclusive.[9]

Alternative medical systems. These are entire systems of belief and practice that represent non-biomedical ways of viewing the body and disease. Examples are traditional Oriental medicine, Ayurvedic medicine, homeopathy, and naturopathy.

Mind-body interventions. These forms of treatment try to evoke the healing powers of the mind to bring about changes in the body. Examples include meditation, some types of hypnosis, and prayer.

Biologically based treatments. These use "natural" products, including herbs, special diets, and supplements, to treat disease. This includes the use of substances such as shark cartilage, laetrile, and bee pollen, as well as vitamins, melatonin, and the like.

Manipulative and body-based methods. These treatments are based on moving various parts of the body. Manipulation of the spine to relieve pain and promote health is especially important in chiropractic and some kinds of osteopathic medicine.

Energy therapies. Practitioners of these therapies believe that energy fields, whether produced naturally by the body or introduced from the outside by magnets, are key to improving health. Schools of practice based on this belief include Reiki and Qi gong.

HYPNOTHERAPY

For decades, many people have looked to hypnosis as a means of strengthening willpower and gaining the upper hand over their cravings and impulses, from compulsive eating to chain smoking. The allure of hypnosis as a possible weapon against overeating is as understandable as is its appeal to many addicted smokers, and for the same reason. If the mind can be "programmed" at some subconscious level,

> **Questions to Ask When Choosing a CAM Practitioner**
>
> Because practitioners of complementary and alternative medicine are often not licensed by the state and not regulated, consumers and patients really need to conduct their own "due diligence." Before ingesting any substance or submitting to any kind of therapy that involves manipulation of your body parts—or any invasive procedure—you need to protect yourself by learning as much as you can about the practice and the practitioner.
>
> Although alternative or natural procedures are often considered by consumers to be benign in comparison with the heavy artillery of modern medicine, such may not be the case. For instance, St. John's wort—a "natural" herb sold widely in grocery stores and pharmacies as an antidote to depression and anxiety—may be dangerous for people who are taking a blood thinner such as coumadin, or who are taking drugs for HIV/AIDS.
>
> The following are some of the recommended questions you should ask before beginning any complementary or alternative therapy:
>
> - What does my regular doctor think about this treatment?
> - Will it conflict with any medicine or medical therapy my doctor is prescribing for me?

maybe we can regain control over desires and appetites that seem to arise without warning and overwhelm our conscious, rational intentions. Many of us may think of a stage magician, or a mesmerizing psychologist with a swinging watch fob when we hear the word "hypnosis." But hypnotherapists themselves describe a process—and a mental state—that is, perhaps, less dramatic to the outward eye, but more meaningful in its long-term consequences. The American Society of Clinical Hypnosis calls hypnosis "a state of inner absorption, concentration and focused attention. It is like using a magnifying glass to focus the rays of the sun and make them more powerful. Similarly, when our minds are concentrated and focused, we are able to

- If not, is it safe and effective in its own right?

- What kind of education and training has this practitioner had? If this practitioner is not in a discipline that is regulated by the state, is he or she a member of a national professional organization that has its own standards of training and accreditation?

- Will this practitioner provide references for me to check out, just like any reputable surgeon?

- How much does this treatment cost, how long will it last, and where will it be delivered? Is the practitioner's office or clinic clean, professional-looking, and readily accessible over the entire course of treatment?

- Will my health insurer pay for the services in question (as might be the case for chiropractic, acupuncture, or massage, for instance) and if so, does my insurance plan require me to use one practitioner or group rather than another to obtain reimbursement?[10]

use our minds more powerfully. Because hypnosis allows people to use more of their potential, learning self-hypnosis is the ultimate act of self-control."[11]

According to the society, hypnosis can be used to treat a variety of diseases and conditions, including pain, skin problems, gastrointestinal problems, and many others, one of which is obesity. However, in choosing a hypnotherapist, the society advises that you look for a licensed health professional—a medical doctor, dentist, psychologist, social worker, therapist, nurse, or other health professional—who is also a member of the American Society of Clinical Hypnosis or the Society for Clinical and Experimental Hypnosis. Similarly, the

American Psychological Association's Division of Psychological Hypnosis declares that hypnosis is not a type of therapy, but rather "a procedure that can be used to facilitate therapy." Therefore, "training in hypnosis is not sufficient for the conduct of therapy. Clinical hypnosis should be used only by properly trained and credentialed health-care professionals . . . who are working within the areas of their professional expertise."[12]

> According to the American Society of Clinical Hypnosis, hypnosis can be used to treat a variety of diseases and conditions, including pain, skin problems, gastrointestinal problems, and many others, one of which is obesity.

While some studies reported in the medical literature suggest a moderate, "adjunctive" role for hypnotherapy in weight control, we suggest that readers be very cautious in responding to advertisements such as the following, featured recently in a Maryland newspaper: "Lose Weight with Hypnosis. 110% Seminar Guarantee." In this advertisement, a self-described hypnotherapist—who lists no credentials as a health professional—promises two "hypnotic sessions" in a seminar for only $39.99. The ad claims that "It's designed so you can lose 30 pounds, 50 pounds, even 120 pounds quickly and safely." Further, the ad says that the seminars have been attended by over 275,000 people, and the program is "designed to work for you just as it has for all these people." How well is that, overall? Of course, the ad does not say. Five people are named, along with the varying impressive amounts of weight they have lost, but an asterisk leading to almost invisible type at the bottom of the ad signals the crucial disclaimer: "Individual results vary."[13]

As indicated previously, some studies have found that hypnotherapy has an add-on effect to other weight-control measures. In one of the relatively few randomized, controlled clinical trials that have been conducted, researchers at Churchill Hospital in Oxford, England, concluded that hypnotherapy produced a statistically meaningful but "small and clinically insignificant" weight loss among obese people suffering from sleep apnea. Of 60 obese people receiving dietary counseling, only the subgroup that also received hypnotherapy aimed at stress reduction was able to maintain a weight loss at 18 months, averaging 3.8 kilograms (about 8 pounds).[14] The researchers concluded that although the effect was modest, further research might be warranted.

Other studies remind us that, like all other forms of treatment, hypnosis may carry its own risks, underlining the advisability of working with licensed health professionals if you decide to go this route. A study of hypnotherapy as a form of weight control for teenagers conducted in the 1970s found that the subjects expected a "quick solution," but for many of the teens—especially those who were less developmentally advanced—it resulted in "severe side effects" including feelings of depersonalization, anxiety, and fears.[15] A 1996 metanalysis (or overview) of six weight-loss studies that compared cognitive-behavioral therapy (counseling) alone to cognitive-behavioral therapy plus hypnotherapy concluded that, at best, hypnotherapy produces a "small enhancement" of weight-loss results.[16]

> Other studies remind us that, like all other forms of treatment, hypnosis may carry its own risks, underlining the advisability of working with licensed health professionals if you decide to go this route.

This is an apt summation of the role of hypnotherapy in weight loss today. Few medical doctors would turn to hypnosis as a primary treatment. Opinions vary on how much it can contribute as a supportive form of therapy. If you decide to give it a try, you would probably be best advised to seek a therapist with formal medical or psychological credentials.

ACUPUNCTURE

Like hypnotherapy, the use of acupuncture for weight loss has many enthusiasts but a limited history of being studied according to the scientific gold standard of randomized, controlled trials. The use of acupuncture in weight loss is, not surprisingly, more widely accepted in China than in the West. In recent years, a number of articles in *The Journal of Traditional Chinese Medicine* have explored this issue. For example, researchers from Chongqing Medical University reported the successful treatment of obesity in 161 people by using a combination of acupressure and acupuncture, claiming that weight had dropped an average of 5 kilograms (11 pounds) in 85 percent of the patients.[17] In another paper, researchers from Nanjing University of Traditional Chinese Medicine reported they had used acupuncture of the body and ear, along with moxibustion (burning of dried herbs on the acupuncture needles) to recontour 359 women who did not suffer from obesity, but had "undesirable body shape." Among other things, the researchers claimed acupuncture could help to regulate BMI, percentage of body fat, chest size, and the ratio of waist to hip.[18]

Obesity is not, however, included in a list of more than 40 conditions for which the World Health Organization views acupuncture as an appropriate form of therapy.[19] Conditions for which it *is* accepted by WHO range from abdominal pain and addiction control to sciatica, sinusitis, and smoking cessation.

> *The use of acupuncture in weight loss is, not surprisingly, more widely accepted in China than in the West.*

In Chinese tradition, the stimulation of more than 2,000 acupuncture points by very fine needles, or by the application of pressure, helps to restore the free flow of the body's natural energy, *qi*, along pathways called *meridians*. To the extent that Western scientists and doctors have accepted acupuncture, they have often interpreted it as somehow triggering the release of certain natural opioids and neurotransmitters, such as endorphins and serotonin, that may relieve pain, stress, and nausea for well-understood biomedical reasons.

Although many Westerners remain skeptical (as we shall discuss below), some medical doctors have adopted acupuncture as a treatment for obesity.

Dr. Richard C. Niemtzow (M.D., Ph.D., MPH), a colonel in the United States Air Force, describes himself as the first full-time acupuncturist in the armed forces. Although he hazards no guess as to its mechanism of action, at least in terms of Western science, he also says there is no doubt that auriculomedicine (acupuncture of the ear) can help obese people lose weight. He says the existence of several important acupuncture points in the ear, including the Appetite Control Point, Shen Men, Point Zero, and Tranquilizer Point, is well documented in the field's literature.

In a recent published study—not a controlled clinical trial—Niemtzow and colleagues at Edwards Air Force Base in California reported using acupuncture of the ear along with a high-protein diet to produce an average weight loss of 19.2 pounds in 43 obese people over a 12-week period. Patients found that the acupuncture treatment had the effect of eliminating their cravings to binge on carbohydrates, the authors reported. They had to be careful lest the acupuncture treatment suppress the appetite too much, as the high-protein diet required participants to eat a sufficient amount of meat. Everyone in the study achieved their weight goals, the paper reported, but telephone follow-up found a relapse rate of 40 percent following discharge.[20] In a personal interview, Dr. Niemtzow explained that he views acupuncture as a very well-studied "alternative technology" that, in the case of obesity and overweight, is useful as a complement to dietary therapy such as the high-protein regimen. He has used acupuncture to treat several hundred people for obesity, but not as a means of weight maintenance after the initial period of weight reduction; for that, he turns patients over to a dietitian, after discussing with them the dietary errors they need to avoid to keep their weight off. "Most people know why they have failed in the past," he said, citing patients who become overweight while eating a pizza for lunch every day and washing it

> *Dr. Niemtzow has used acupuncture to treat several hundred people for obesity, but not as a means of weight maintenance after the initial period of weight reduction; for that, he turns patients over to a dietitian, after discussing with them the dietary errors they need to avoid to keep their weight off.*

down with a quart of soda pop. Acupuncture will not prevent overeaters from regaining their weight if they revert to their old ways. Thus it is likely that the acupuncture, like hypnosis, is only an adjunct to standard treatment. In no instance can it be said that weight loss using these adjunctive techniques is due to anything other than the fact that food consumption is diminished temporarily, perhaps as a result of the patient's belief that the adjunctive treatment works.

A slightly different tack to treating obesity is being taken by acupuncturist Dean Richards in Australia. Richards has developed an ear clip called AcuSlim that draws on a battery pack to administer a slight electric current to the acupuncture points. AcuSlim's manufacturer, S.H.P. International Pty. Ltd., quoting published research by Richards, claims that the device stimulates a branch of the vagal nerve, raising serotonin and dopamine levels in the body and serving to "increase tone in the smooth muscles of the stomach, thus suppressing appetite."[21] The technique is described as a form of transcutaneous electric nerve simulation (TENS), similar to a procedure that has produced pain relief in some people suffering from chronic back pain. In a published paper with a University of Adelaide researcher, Richards reported on the results of a controlled study. Sixty overweight people were divided into two groups with the goal of losing 2 kilograms (4.4 pounds) in 4 weeks. One group used the ear clip twice a day for 4 weeks, whereas those in the other (control group) simply attached the clip to their thumbs, which are inert, acupuncturally speaking. Ninety-five percent of those who wore the clip on their ears (the "active" group) reported their appetites diminished, whereas none in the control group did, and none in the control group met the relatively modest weight-loss goal. Ninety-three percent of the active group, however, lost weight, and more than three-quarters met the 4-pound goal.[22]

> *Ninety-five percent of those who wore the clip on their ears reported their appetites diminished, whereas none in the control group did.*

Although popular interest in acupuncture as a weight-control measure is keen—Niemtzow says he gets calls about the subject from around the country almost every day—much of the medical community is unconvinced. A 1999 randomized, controlled trial at the University of Florence in Italy divided 40 obese patients into two groups. One group received acupuncture of the ear along with moxibustion, or burning of herbs, whereas the other received minimal acupuncture of the body (placebo). Both groups were measured before and after the 12-week trial to determine their BMIs and their psychological attributes of anxiety, depression, and attitudes toward eating. The upshot? The group getting the "real" acupuncture treatment improved substantially with regard to anxiety and depression. But neither group achieved significant weight loss.[23] Similarly, an English researcher's review of four published clinical trials on acupuncture and acupressure and their effects on weight loss found they all had "methodological flaws," came to contradictory conclusions, and formed "no clear picture" of weight reduction.[24] An American surgeon, reviewing dozens of failed procedures for weight control, listed acupuncture as a "questionable" treatment for obesity along with many abandoned gastric surgery techniques, liposuction, and tooth wiring.[25]

An American surgeon, reviewing dozens of failed procedures for weight control, listed acupuncture as a "questionable" treatment for obesity along with many abandoned gastric surgery techniques, liposuction, and tooth wiring.

A humorous postscript to this area of investigation was provided in an online chat on the Web site of the American Academy of Medical Acupuncture. Asked whether he had any "new pearls" to suggest on the subject of obesity, Dr. Jeff Baird, an acupuncturist, responded, "There is none. Acupuncture works as well as anything for addressing cravings until the person can make some lifestyle changes, but it won't replace it. As our master used to say, if acupuncture worked for obesity, there wouldn't be so many fat acupuncturists."[26]

NONPRESCRIPTION DRUGS

Along with the bulging national waistline has come a growing number of nonprescription (over-the-counter) diet pills and food supplements. A visit to almost any grocery or drug store will reveal shelves full of these dietary aids, whose purchase is part of the more than $33 billion a year the government estimates Americans spend on weight loss or weight-prevention products and services.[27] At any given time, about one-quarter of American men and nearly 40 percent of American women say they are trying to lose weight. Nonprescription diet aids have proliferated as manufacturers scramble to meet this demand. Sales of herbal supplements have remained steady in recent years at about $4 billion.[28]

The fact that you can buy over-the-counter drugs and diet aids without a doctor's prescription does not mean that they can be taken without thought, like candy (the same holds true for "natural" herbs—which are, in fact, among these diet aids' most important ingredients). Read the manufacturer's label carefully. You will find that even these products can result in high blood pressure, nervousness, sleeplessness, and other unpleasant side effects if they are used at excessive dosages or for longer than the recommended periods of time. Some of these drugs are not recommended for use by people under 18. Most important, from a doctor's perspective, is that these drugs will not bring about either dramatic or long-lasting weight loss.

> *The fact that you can buy over-the-counter drugs and diet aids without a doctor's prescription does not mean that they can be taken without thought, like candy.*

If you read all the fine print, you will see the disclaimer saying that the product in question is not intended to prevent, treat, or cure any disease, and that the manufacturer's statements about it have not been evaluated by the Food and Drug Administration. Rather, these products are produced and sold under the terms of the Dietary Supplement Health and Education Act of 1994 (DSHEA), which gave manufacturers of nutritional supplements wide latitude in introducing and marketing new preparations as long as they do not claim that they treat disease. Dietary supplements as defined by the act include vitamins, minerals, herbs, other botanical (plant) substances, amino acids, and other items intended to increase dietary intake. The FDA steps in only after the fact in extraordinary circumstances, such as when there are reports of injury or death, or manufacturers make disease-treatment claims that go beyond what is legally permissible. Therefore, consumers cannot assume that these preparations have undergone the same extensive testing for safety and effectiveness that is true of FDA-regulated pharmaceuticals prescribed for them by their doctors. You are truly on your own when you buy and use these preparations. This is one case when you *must* read the fine print and be aware of what you are doing. *Caveat emptor*—buyer beware—applies particularly to these products because they have generally not been subjected to anywhere near the amount of testing for safety and effectiveness that prescription medicines, or even over-the-counter (OTC) medicines, are required to undergo.

> Consumers cannot assume that these preparations have undergone the same extensive testing for safety and effectiveness that is true of FDA-regulated pharmaceuticals prescribed for them by their doctors. You are truly on your own when you buy and use these preparations.

Ephedrine

A reading of the label of Dexatrim Natural Green Tea Formula, one of the dozens of OTC products freely available to any shopper in many pharmacies and grocery stores, will reveal that at the essence of this diet aid are two drugs, neither of which is regulated by the FDA—caffeine and ephedrine.[29] Ephedrine is a powerful stimulant that is related both to methamphetamines and phenylpropanolamine (PPA), an ingredient in both cold medicines and diet aids that was withdrawn from the market at the request of the FDA in 2000 after a

Yale University study linked it to a heightened risk of hemorrhagic stroke. Dexatrim's manufacturer recommends taking two caplets per day, amounting to 24 milligrams of ephedrine, and states that the maximum recommended dosage of ephedrine is 100 milligrams per day for no more than 12 weeks.

The company also warns that the product is not intended for people who are pregnant or nursing a baby; who suffer from heart disease, diabetes, or a wide variety of other illnesses; or who are using certain other prescription and nonprescription drugs. The product should not be used by people under 18 and cannot legally be sold to people 17 and under in Texas. The company warns that "exceeding recommended serving may cause serious adverse health effects, including heart attack and stroke." Users should call a doctor immediately if they experience dizziness, rapid heartbeat, severe headache "or other similar symptoms."

Several things about this are worthy of comment. First, these are not idle warnings. All of the company's cautions, and recommended dosage limits, should be followed scrupulously if you choose to use diet aids. Second, note the 12-week limit. Even if this product works as advertised for you, 3 months is not a long time compared to the rest of your life. You are going to have to make permanent lifestyle changes to keep off any weight you might lose. And finally, pay special attention to the warnings against use of this drug by anyone suffering from heart disease or diabetes. Obviously, many very obese people suffer from these very conditions, and may or may not be aware that they have these conditions.

Although the FDA's ability to regulate dietary supplements is limited under the terms of the DSHEA, it has collected hundreds of reports of serious illness—and some deaths—among ephedra users since 1993, when it established a voluntary consumer-reporting hotline. Consumers can report problems involving any drug or dietary supplement online at www.accessdata.fda.gov/scripts/medwatch, or by calling (888) INFO-FDA or (301) 443-1240.

The FDA has proposed regulations that establish dosage limits for ephedra but has not, to date, received permission to implement them. The Dexatrim green tea's 24-milligram daily dosage falls within the FDA's recommended dosage limit. However, the recommended 12-week time limit does not. The FDA proposed labeling that would have limited the use of ephedra to 7 days; opposed any claims for its effectiveness—such as bodybuilding or weight loss—that would have required users to take it for longer periods of time; and opposed combinations of the drug with caffeine or other stimulants, as frequently occurs in diet aids.[30] Today ephedra remains one of the most commonly found active ingredients in over-the-counter diet aids, including Herbalife and Metabolife. You may see the same ingredient referred to as *ma huang* (its Chinese name), Chinese ephedra, Ephedra Sinica, Sida Cordifolia or epitonin.

> Consumers can report problems involving any drug or dietary supplement online at www.accessdata.fda.gov/scripts/medwatch, or by calling (888) INFO-FDA or (301) 443-1240.

Ephedra remains controversial, with the FDA under pressure from anti-ephedra groups such as the consumer group Public Citizen on the one hand, and pro-ephedra industry groups on the other. Ephedra makers say that the supplement is safe if consumers observe the label warnings and do not exceed recommended dosage limits. Public Citizen petitioned the FDA to ban ephedra-containing products in September 2001, saying the FDA's own database shows it has received more than 1,300 reports of adverse reactions to ephedra, including 81 deaths.[31] A few months earlier, Health Canada, a government agency, issued a public advisory warning Canadians not to use ephedra either alone or in combination with stimulants such as caffeine. In addition to reports of deaths and injury collected by the U.S. FDA, Health Canada said it had received 60 reports of serious illness that may have been connected to the use of dietary supplements containing ephedra.[32]

The fact is, ephedrine is arguably the only effective ingredient available either over the counter or in herbal preparations for appetite control. It is likely that any effectiveness of OTCs and herbals is due primarily or solely to this agent. Used in recommended doses for short periods, with attention paid to the warnings, it is likely about as effective and generally safe as prescribed appetite suppressants, which act in similar ways. Combinations of ephedra with caffeine and other ephedra-containing compounds, such as some decongestants, is inadvisable, especially without medical supervision.

> *Ephedra remains controversial, with the FDA under pressure from anti-ephedra groups such as the consumer group Public Citizen on the one hand, and pro-ephedra industry groups on the other.*

Fat Magnets

Another highly promoted "natural" fat fighter is chitosan, a substance derived from a hard material called chitin in the shells of crustaceans, including crabs, lobsters, and shrimp. Chitin is even more ubiquitous in nature than the cellulose found in plants.[33] Enthusiasts of chitosan claim, in effect, that it has some of the same properties as Xenical (orlistat)—that it latches onto fatty acids in the human digestive system and prevents them from being absorbed, thus passing through the body without adding any calories or pounds. Hence, you may often see chitosan-containing pills advertised as Fat Magnets, Fat Trappers, and similar names.

Although there is no compelling evidence that chitosan performs as claimed in humans, it would have many of the same side effects as orlistat if it did—meaning that users would need to take vitamin supplements to replace fat-soluble vitamins leached from their bodies. In one animal study, rats eating large doses of chitosan for 2 weeks experienced a sharp drop in the vitamin E levels in their blood. A 1997 study of mice found that a diet high in chitosan led to a decline in the number of certain naturally occurring—and beneficial—bacteria in their intestines.[34]

Whether it's worth these theoretical risks is, in our minds, an easy question to answer. Chitosan has not proven that it can do the job its promoters claim. In one study, 12 volunteers took either orlistat or chitosan for 7 days. They then switched, taking the other treatment for the next 7 days. Their stools were collected in days 4 to 7 of each study period so that their excretion of fat could be measured. The study showed that their excretion of fat increased "significantly" with orlistat, but not with chitosan.[35] In another randomized, double-blind trial, researchers in the Department of Complementary Medicine of the University of Exeter in England found chitosan had no significant effect on the Body Mass Index, cholesterol, or triglycerides of overweight volunteers who took it, as compared with those who took a placebo for four weeks.[36]

Though a product such as chitosan may seem basically harmless, if ineffective, some of the advertising and marketing practices used to hawk it to the American public have been particularly egregious. In April 2000, the Federal Trade Commission won a $10 million judgment from a federal court in California against Enforma Natural Product, Inc. Enforma promoted its chitosan-based "Fat Trapper" and another product, "Exercise in a Bottle," in 30-minute infomercials starring former major-league baseball player Steve Garvey. The FTC said the company could not substantiate its claims that Fat Trapper "permanently" blocks fat, and that "Exercise in a Bottle works on a cellular level, forcing every cell in your body to work, whether you're exercising or not. And when your cells are working, you are burning calories or losing fat."[37] The company had assured users that its system "helps your body to burn more calories while you're just standing or sitting around doing nothing—even while you're sleeping." The "Exercise in a Bottle" notion was based on an ingredient known as pyruvate, which is a chemical formed when the body metabolizes (or burns) food. Proponents claim that pyruvate promotes thermogenesis, or the conversion of more calories to heat rather than to their storage in the form of fat. However, there

> *Whether it's worth these theoretical risks is, in our minds, an easy question to answer. Chitosan has not proven that it can do the job its promoters claim.*

> **A Cautionary Tale**
>
> Though desperate weight-watchers usually have little more to lose than their spare cash, that is not always the worst that may happen.
>
> In 2000, the FDA issued an alert to consumers to not use any botanical products containing aristolochic acid, found in a variety of herbal medicines and traditional Chinese medicines. The agency cited cases of severe kidney disease leading to renal dialysis and the need for kidney transplant in Belgium, France, England, and the United States.
>
> In one particularly shocking episode, 70 patients at a Belgian weight-loss clinic who had taken an herbal product containing aristolochic acid suffered kidney failure. Moreover, 18 of them were diagnosed with a rare form of cancer of the urinary tract, thought to be related to their use of the same herbal product.

is little or no convincing evidence that pyruvate works as claimed or that it is safe when taken for any extended period of time.

Other Questionable "Diet Aids"

In recent years, the FDA has also cautioned consumers against misuse and the possible dangers of "dieter's teas," many containing stimulant laxatives that may promote quick but temporary loss of water weight. Because calories are absorbed in the small intestine, not in the colon where these teas achieve their effects, their efficacy is highly suspect. The FDA said that four deaths of young women may have been linked to these teas, which contained herbal ingredients such as senna, aloe, and buckthorn.[38]

Remarkably, anyone who has access to the Internet, or who reads popular magazines, will have no trouble finding exaggerated weight-

> A woman in the United States developed end-stage renal disease—a form of kidney failure requiring lifelong dialysis or transplant—only 8 months after beginning to use herbal medicines, the FDA said, and a second patient developed the same condition after 2 years of taking a botanical product that may have contained aristolochic acid (despite a label identifying it as another herb).
>
> The FDA warned consumers against taking the following products, all of which contain aristolochic acid:
>
> Rheumixx; BioSlim Doctor's Natural Weight Loss System Slim Tone Formula; Prostatin; Fang Ji Stephania; Mu Tong *Clematis armandi;* Temple of Heaven Chinese Herbs Radix aristolochiae; Meridian Circulation; Qualiherb Chinese Herbal Formulas Dianthus Formulas Ba Zheng San; Clematis & Carthamus Formula 21280; Virginia Snake Root, Cut, *Aristolochia serpentaria;* Green Kingdom Akebia Extract; Green Kingdom Stephania Extract; Neo Concept Aller Relief.[39]

loss claims today. Thus a full-page ad, for instance, for the apple-pectin-based "Quick Slim Fat Blocker" in a popular magazine (*Us Weekly*, October 1, 2001) promises 2-pound-a-day weight loss, "without diet or exercise." A bulk e-mail for the "all-natural Growth Hormone therapy supplements" promises "truly incredible" benefits, including decreased body fat, increased lean muscle mass, and "easy" weight loss. A mass fax which appeared overnight (August 15, 2001) in one of our home offices purports to "Safely Eliminate Fat Forever, Without Diet." The company, Nutri-Pro, says that its new breakthrough weight-management system, "Ultra-Perfect," combines Ultra Pyruvate and another product, the Fat Absorber, which "does the hard work while your body burns the stored fat for energy." Though the names and labels change, the underlying concepts begin to fall into a recognizable pattern for the thoughtful consumer. Unfortunately, if you think it sounds too good to be true, you are correct.

SUMMARY

Because medical science has not offered simple and effective solutions to reverse the tide of obesity, many people, understandably, are looking for alternative treatments. These treatments range from the relatively exotic (acupuncture, hypnotherapy) to the relatively familiar ("natural" herbs and teas) that can be brewed or swallowed. Though some small weight-loss effects have been documented for some of these alternative modalities, by and large, they have not passed muster with rigorous controlled studies in which their effects were compared with those of a placebo not known to either the researchers or the volunteer participants. Many weight-loss treatments—whether they are real alternative forms of therapy or harmless placebos—work for a while for a very simple reason: The volunteers want them to. Therefore, they pay special attention to how much they eat and how much exercise they get.

> *Remarkably, anyone who has access to the Internet or who reads popular magazines, will have no trouble finding exaggerated weight-loss claims today.*

Although many forms of treatment are harmless, if ineffective, some can be damaging to your health. It is important to consult your doctor before beginning any alternative therapy—even "natural" weight-loss pills you might think are safe because you get them in your grocery store or pharmacy. In fact, thanks to a 1994 law passed by Congress, if these products are marketed only as dietary supplements rather than drugs, their safety and effectiveness has *not* been evaluated by the Food and Drug Administration. And many of these herbal products may interact with prescription drugs you are already taking.

If you've tried some of these nonprescription treatments, you're not alone. Based on telephone interviews of nearly 15,000 adults, researchers from the Centers for Disease Control and Prevention estimated that 17 million Americans used nonprescription weight-loss products from 1996 to 1998. Use of these products was more common among women than men, and especially among young, obese women, more than one-fourth of whom had gone this route. The researchers concluded that advising their patients on the use of dietary supplements (and alternative weight-control treatments generally) will be a growing challenge for doctors.[40] There are more and more products on the market all the time, and most all of them have *not* been tested in a scientifically sound way. We believe the use of alternative drug products should be viewed with the same skepticism with which so many people view prescription drugs—they have the potential to be just as dangerous, and what's worse, have not been required to undergo the careful, scientific testing that prescription drugs must undergo. Due to the fact that there are often problems with prescription drugs that are discovered later—even after all the safety and efficacy testing—resulting in them being withdrawn from the market, it should be clear that the risks from untested, unregulated herbal drugs and supplements will be that much greater. We caution you not to be lulled into a false sense of security because a product is labeled "natural" or "herbal." Most poisons are also of herbal origin, and all plants contain drugs and chemicals just as surely as a pharmaceutical company's factory does.

> *Many weight-loss treatments—whether they are real alternative forms of therapy or harmless placebos—work for a while for a very simple reason: The volunteers want them to.*

CHAPTER 7

Family, Society, and Our Overweight Kids

OBESITY BEGINS AT home. That simple truism reflects the fact that obesity stems from a multitude of biological, cultural, social, and psychological factors, all of which have their roots, for most of us, at home—in our families of origin. Home is where we get our genes. Remember that up to 30 to 50 percent of the variances in body fat between people are believed to be due to their genes—and by one recent count, up to 130 genes or gene markers may be involved.[1] Home is also where we learn to eat—what to eat, how much to eat, and how often to eat. For that reason, home is the very place where most obese people develop an unhealthy relationship with food while they are still children, learning the rules for how to use and abuse mealtime and snack time alike, without even being fully conscious of the lessons they are absorbing.

Yet obesity is not confined to home. It has a public dimension and takes on its larger meaning in relation to society as a whole. The obese person acts and interacts in a culture that often judges and stereotypes the overweight. This is true even though, paradoxically, the number of overweight and obese people is at an all-time high in the history of the human race. Fortunately, as awareness of the medical dimensions of obesity has grown, some advances have been made in laws and regulations that are favorable to those who are overweight. We will discuss them later in this chapter.

For many obese people, their condition also has strong and undeniable psychological components. The act of eating and the emotional significance of food take on certain roles and meanings that should instead be played out with other people, perhaps, or through recreational activities. As Linda Cartwright, the woman profiled in chapter 2, reported, food was a way of making herself feel more powerful when her father threatened her mother. It helped her get larger; if she could only get larger, she thought, she would be safe. She also confessed that food was a dependable way of obtaining solace at the end of a day when she was lonely; given different circumstances, she would rather have been intimate with a spouse.

> *Obesity is not confined to home. It has a public dimension and takes on its larger meaning in relation to society as a whole.*

For many others, food is a response to stress—stress on the job, stress after an argument with one's spouse or child, even stress about feeling oneself growing heavier. A dependable way to stave off those gnawing feelings of anxiety is to reach for a pint of ice cream or a bag of chips—even if you know, intellectually, that you may be feeding one of the problems that made you feel stressed in the first place. Reason has little to do with this set of behaviors, which is why changing a lifetime of actions and reactions for many people requires a support group with professional leadership and a long-term commitment.

Beginning in the teen years, home for many people is where eating disorders first manifest themselves. By now, almost everyone is familiar with the terms *anorexia nervosa* and *bulimia nervosa*. Increasingly, doctors recognize the category of binge eating disorders as being in this group. While technically binge eating disorders and obesity are different, they may overlap in up to one-quarter of obese people.[2] That can be especially true of nighttime binge eating disorders, which can lead some people to consume more than half the day's calories after everyone else in their family has finished dinner. Since food eaten this late almost by definition is not going to be burned to support physical activity prior to sleep, nighttime binge eating is very likely to contribute to weight gain.

Anyone who treats obese individuals—especially those who are morbidly obese—knows that a high percentage of them are depressed. What almost no one can say with confidence, however, is whether the depression has caused the obesity or the obesity has led to the depression. Whichever way the lines of causation run, there definitely is an association, and it gets greater in proportion to the degree of obesity.

> *What almost no one can say with confidence is whether the depression has caused the obesity or the obesity has led to the depression.*

Finally, a bitter and unpleasant fact discovered by many doctors in the course of treating severely obese patients is that many of them were physically, emotionally, or sexually abused as children. One mentions this point with some qualms. It would be extremely unfair—and inaccurate—to say that all, or even most, clinically obese people are victims of childhood abuse. Yet undeniably, for a significant minority, this is an issue that surfaces.

We shall discuss these psychological issues before turning to the related and extremely important issues of society's treatment of the obese and childhood obesity.

PSYCHOLOGICAL ISSUES

Perhaps the first and, in this context, most important point to make about overweight and obesity is that they are not forms of mental illness. Although eating disorders are classified as mental disorders in the *Diagnostic and Statistical Manual of Mental Disorders*, obesity is not. Obesity can be the result of a multitude of different physical and behavioral factors, rather than a mental illness. Remember those 130-odd different genes, which can express themselves in such wildly variant ways as a propensity to "fidget," thus burning calories while resting, or a biochemical predilection for turning high-fat meals to adipose tissue? A few of these genetically linked conditions may be characterized as illnesses (see chapter 1), while many others reflect simple differences between individuals. Researcher Richard L. Atkinson of the University of Wisconsin speculates that there may be, literally, "thousands of different types of obesity," reflecting the vast number of different gene combinations that may be present in any given individual.[3]

> Obese people display all the infinite variety of personality and character traits that characterize those of "normal" weight.

Researchers have studied the psychology of obese people for decades and have failed to discover any particular kind of psychiatric illness that characterizes the overweight and obese. Rather, obese people display all the infinite variety of personality and character traits that characterize those of "normal" weight.

Researchers Donald Williamson and Patrick O'Neil, reviewing the published literature on obesity and psychology, say that no "obese personality" exists. "It appears that the obese differ from each other as much as they differ from non-obese people, on psychological characteristics and traits not explicitly concerned with weight and eating," they write. "Indeed, given the vast numbers of obese people, it would be naive to expect otherwise." However, when it comes to characteristics specifically related to food, eating, weight, and body image, important differences do emerge. Obese people are more likely to be depressed and have self-defeating thoughts and attitudes when it comes to issues of weight control and eating. Obese people, both in and out of clinical settings, also are more liable to report "difficulty in controlling negative emotional eating, food temptations, and overeating," and they tend to score higher on a standard test used to evaluate people's perceptions of their own hunger, Williamson and O'Neil report.[4] Some of this may strike you as science vindicating common sense. But it also corresponds well with our experience at the Johns Hopkins Weight Management Center. The more obese individuals are, the more likely they are to be depressed. Also, the more likely they are to report frequently eating not in response to physical symptoms of hunger but when they encounter such everyday triggers as boredom, unease, stress, or depression. Of course, this pattern can become a vicious, self-perpetuating cycle. The more we shovel in the "comfort food," the less pleased we may be with changes in our appearance and health. The more we possibly worsen any physical symptoms associated with overweight, the more comfort we may need. And given the fact that clinical obesity commonly leads to decreased mobility, increased pain, and poor quality of sleep—not to mention diabetes, heart disease, and social stigma—it is not surprising to encounter more and more signs and symptoms of depression as people grow heavier.

> *The more we shovel in the "comfort food," the less pleased we may be with changes in our appearance and health.*

The flip side of this coin, of course, is that obese people often experience steady improvement in many aspects of their emotional, physical, and psychological functioning as they are able to lose weight and achieve a sense of self-mastery.

Eating Disorders and Obesity

As noted earlier, obesity is not defined by the psychiatric profession as an eating disorder or as a mental illness. While not as common as overweight and obesity, eating disorders, in contrast, are viewed as psychiatric illnesses—illnesses that revolve around food, body image, and eating behavior. Moreover, as we shall see, there is some overlap between obesity and at least one form of eating disorder.

Anorexia Nervosa

Anorexia nervosa, perhaps the most famous eating disorder because it claimed the life of singer Karen Carpenter and is a particular risk for highly trained ballerinas and gymnasts, is relatively rare but is believed by many to be on the increase. About 95 percent of anorexics are female, and those in middle-class or upper-middle-class income brackets are more likely to be affected. A study of teenage girls in London during the 1970s estimated 1 in every 200 were severely anorexic.[5] Other studies have found the incidence to be rising from decade to decade.

The very antithesis of obesity, anorexia is marked by the fear and loathing of becoming fat. The anorexic's self-image may be warped, leading to an inability to accept normal weight, along with an obsession with remaining rail-thin. Many authors have observed that anorexia is an exaggerated reaction to cover-girl stereotypes that define feminine beauty in the entertainment media as well as in the world of high fashion. Anorexics can either practice severe caloric restriction by not eating, or indulge in the binge-and-purge behavior of gorging themselves and then vomiting, as seen in bulimics. They suffer from a variety of physical ailments including electrolyte disturbances (recall the discussion of Very Low Calorie Diets, which must be medically supervised for that reason, among others), heightened vulnerability to infections, and low bone density. A stunningly high 5 to 7 percent of people with anorexia die within 10 years.[6]

> *Anorexics can either practice severe caloric restriction by not eating, or indulge in the binge-and-purge behavior of gorging themselves and then vomiting, as seen in bulimics.*

Anorexics, perhaps not surprisingly, are often found also to have anxiety, depression, and obsessive-compulsive disorder, or the irrational repetition of rituals that have personal meaning. At least one researcher has found that the *mothers* of anorexics are more likely to display obsessive-compulsive tendencies than a control group of women the same age, while others have found a heightened tendency to anorexia in first- and second-degree relatives of anorexics, as compared with the population at large. Some speculate that this observation enforces the possibility of a family-linked biological imbalance in a brain hormone called *serotonin*, which helps regulate appetite and mood.[7]

Bulimia Nervosa

Bulimia nervosa is much more frequent, with an occurrence estimated at 4 to 9 percent of the high school and college-age population in some studies. Bulimia, from the Greek word for "ox hunger," refers to a syndrome in which people gorge themselves with food—called *binge eating*—but then also take compensatory measures to keep themselves from gaining weight. Like anorexia, bulimia is overwhelmingly a disorder of young women, though men are more likely to be bulimic than anorexic. Sports that emphasize weight control, especially wrestling, in which participants must make a weight limit to stay in their class, may foster bulimia in young men, just as ballet, ice skating, and gymnastics may do in young women. The first appearance of bulimia almost always follows a period of dieting.[8] Bulimics can use laxatives, induce vomiting, or engage in fasting or excessive exercise to purge the great amounts of food they can pack into their bodies in short periods of time.

> Bulimics can use laxatives, induce vomiting, or engage in fasting or excessive exercise to purge the great amounts of food they can pack into their bodies in short periods of time.

Unlike anorexics, bulimics are not morbidly thin and therefore have a lower risk of death. However, the bulimic's abuse of emetic syrup of ipecac to induce vomiting can lead to death from cardiomyopathy, or long-term weakening of the heart. Habitual vomiting can also lead to electrolyte imbalances followed by cardiac arrhythmias and possible death.[9] Bulimics frequently consume several thousand calories' worth of food in just 1 or 2 hours; as clinically defined, this behavior is accompanied by a feeling of being out of control, which is then followed by feelings of guilt and shame.

Psychological studies have found that people suffering from bulimia also often have problems with poor impulse control, which can lead to heightened rates of alcoholism and substance abuse, shoplifting, and sexual promiscuity. Bulimics have a heightened rate of depression when compared to the general population. As with anorexia, researchers suspect possible disturbances of the hormone serotonin, a neurotransmitter involved in regulating mood, appetite, and impulsivity.[10] As with many biochemical alterations suspected of causing disease, though, it is difficult to distinguish between abnormalities that are a consequence of the disease itself (for example, chronic vomiting in and of itself might lead to serotonin abnormalities) and primary abnormalities that lead to a disease. Only further studies will establish whether a causal connection exists.

Binge Eating Disorder

Binge eating disorder has been recognized in recent years as a syndrome that is distinct from bulimia nervosa. Like bulimics, people with binge eating disorder can pile on calories by the thousands in brief, intense bouts of eating. The episodes must occur an average of at least twice a week for 6 months to be classified as binge eating disorder. Unlike bulimics, those with binge eating disorder do not attempt to compensate by purging the food from their bodies. The consequences over time are obvious. About 8 percent of all obese people, and up to 30 percent of obese people seeking medical treatment for their obesity, have been found to suffer from binge eating disorder, meaning binge eating may be anywhere from 4 to 15 times more common among the obese than in the population at large.[11] Italian researchers interviewing more than 90 "massively obese" individuals preparing for bariatric surgery found that more than half of them were binge eaters.[12] Thus, the rate of binge eating appears to increase as people become more obese.

> *Unlike bulimics, those who suffer from binge eating disorder do not attempt to compensate by purging the food from their bodies.*

As for what we can expect for people who engage in binge eating, the outcome resembles that of bulimia—or obesity itself. In one study of 68 such people, individuals who were treated as inpatients (and thus likely a more seriously ill population of binge eaters than average), about 57 percent had a "good outcome," 35 percent an "intermediate outcome," 6 percent a "poor outcome," and 1.4 percent died.[13]

As with bulimia, binge eating disorder seems to be associated with a heightened risk of other forms of psychological disorder, such as depression, impulsivity, borderline personality disorder, and substance abuse. But careful research has been able to tease apart binge eating disorder from obesity; the two must not be equated. "Among obese individuals, the presence of binge eating disorder may explain the increased levels of psychopathology previously attributed to the presence of obesity per se," writes National Institutes of Health researcher Susan Yanovski.[14]

Night Eating Syndrome

Some researchers have urged the recognition of yet another eating disorder that may be strongly associated with obesity in some people—*night eating syndrome*. Researchers at the New York Obesity Research Center say night eating syndrome deserves recognition as a distinct disorder with an especially poor prognosis with respect to the ability to lose weight. People who have this syndrome tend to skip

---

One Theory Dashed

Because eating disorders frequently are noticed in young people, especially in young women, after attempts at dieting, some have wondered whether dieting in older, obese people might lead to the development of eating disorders. Recently, the National Task Force on the Prevention and Treatment of Obesity reviewed a number of published studies bearing on this issue and found little evidence to support this theory. Losing weight, or preventing further weight gain, has more positive than negative psychological effects for most overweight people, the task force concluded. To reap the benefit of weight loss means eating less—restricting calories by dieting—along with increasing levels of physical activity.[15]

breakfast four or more days per week, typically eat more than half of their calories after 7 P.M., and report difficulty sleeping on four or more nights per week. Those falling into this category tended to be more depressed and have lower self-esteem than a control group, the researchers reported.[16]

How Are Eating Disorders Treated?

Treatment plans vary but typically include medical evaluation and treatment, consultations with a registered dietitian, psychological therapy, group support or self-help sessions with peers, and drug therapy. Drug therapy can be aimed at alleviating symptoms associated with anxiety, depression, or obsessive-compulsive disorder, if they are present. Doctors who specialize in eating disorders say they can be difficult to treat and require patience and time. Experience shows that 85 percent of individuals with anorexia nervosa can regain their lost weight during inpatient treatment in a hospital or clinic, but 50 to 60 percent relapse after 1 year, says Dr. L. K. George Hsu, a Boston psychiatrist. Denial that anything is wrong and sabotage of the treatment plan by the person with anorexia are often encountered.[17]

> *Doctors who specialize in eating disorders say they can be difficult to treat and require patience and time.*

Because binge eating disorder is a fairly new classification, not many long-term studies of treatment outcomes for people with this condition have been done yet. However, generally prescribed treatment involves psychotherapy and the use of antidepressants.

Stress and Obesity

No doubt for many people, because of the emotional meanings of food, stress is one of the triggers that often leads to eating in the absence of real physical hunger. And this response, in turn, leads to weight gain. Keeping a food journal, as discussed in chapter 3, can help you identify the situations and episodes in your life that have you reaching for the cookie jar or a pint of ice cream. Over time, patterns will emerge that help you identify your reaction to stress, and you will be able to respond to stress in more healthful ways. You may find, for instance, that arguments with the kids about doing their homework after dinner leave you upset and reaching for a second helping of dessert, just to calm your nerves. Believe it or not, experience and clinical evidence show that if you can distract yourself for only 15 to 20 minutes when you feel an urge to eat at an inappropriate time, the urge will often pass. Then, the next time you feel a hunger pang, it will be more likely to represent a real need to eat, as opposed to a conditioned response to some other negative emotion (or to a food trigger on TV).

> *It is often literally true that a walk around the block will help you get past the impulse to snack at an inappropriate time.*

Thus, it is often literally true that a walk around the block will help you get past the impulse to snack at an inappropriate time. It will be doubly good for you, too, in that the exercise actually will burn some calories and increase your muscle tone. As to how to get your kids to do their homework on time—well, that's another book!

Child Abuse and Obesity

As mentioned earlier, many obese people have suffered sexual, physical, or emotional abuse as children. This statement does *not* mean that most obese people have been abused or that we should automatically perceive an obese person as a victim of child abuse. Nevertheless, for those who treat obese people, this factor is one of the ingredients that lead to sympathy, understanding, and the need for professional counseling whenever abuse is found to be present in the medical history. Keep in mind, however, that a history of abuse does not always come out in an initial interview.

Reliable statistics are understandably scarce in this extremely sensitive area. In one study of 145 people diagnosed with binge eating disorder, Yale psychiatrists found that fully 83 percent said they had been abused or maltreated as children—with 59 percent reporting emotional abuse, 36 percent reporting physical abuse, and 30 percent reporting sexual abuse. However, there was no systematic link between any given type of abuse and the Body Mass Index (or relative degree of obesity) in these people.[18]

Families and Sabotage

We began this chapter by observing that obesity begins at home. Often, it is perpetuated at home as well. In the weight-management profession, we call that sort of perpetuation *sabotage*. It is remarkable how often people tell us that those around them—often their husbands, but sometimes others, such as their parents—undercut their efforts to get serious about a weight-control program. This behavior may be innocent and well intended. A man who knows his wife likes chocolates, for instance, may get in the habit of bringing a box home to please her. But after the wife has passed 200 pounds, this formerly endearing gesture is not so benign anymore. Her protests—particularly when she has begun to concentrate on changing her food environment, as well as rescripting her own emotional triggers that lead to overeating—may get a wide-eyed response: "Well, if you don't want them, just don't eat them. They're here if you want a treat."

> *The strategies will vary depending on your relationship with the person who is tempting (or tormenting) you, the communication styles the two of you have developed, and the degree of motivation and self-insight the other person can achieve while you are going through your weight-control program.*

Over time, we try to help people develop strategies to deal with their own spouses or families on issues like this one. The strategies will vary depending on your relationship with the person who is tempting (or tormenting) you, the communication styles the two of you have developed, and the degree of motivation and self-insight the other person can achieve while you are going through your weight-control program.

Some types of sabotage, of course, represent conscious attempts at control. For people locked in relationships with a controlling mate, professional counseling is warranted.

Needless to say, many people are threatened by significant change, whether in themselves or in their family members. They may be afraid that a newly slender partner will not love them anymore or will be more attractive to others. Any or all of these issues can come into play and must be discussed, understood, and managed as part of a long-term weight-management strategy. The issues comprising sabotage are yet another reason why long-term peer support groups, led by a knowledgeable professional, can be important to many people who are trying to introduce lasting change into their lives by losing weight.

At a basic level, of course, families can also be critical to weight control if the frequency, schedule, and composition of meals served in the home are inappropriate. A mother, spouse, or caregiver who resists changes in the way she or he cooks to accommodate the needs of an obese person can make life—and shedding extra pounds—difficult. This is especially true if the obese person has been labeled as the "fat one" since childhood. Most people, of course, respond well to education. But make no mistake, a certain degree of reeducation or retraining of all concerned in the family unit will be critical. Long-term success at weight control will hinge on the ability of the obese person to change not only him- or herself but also wide-reaching webs of interaction with surrounding intimates. This usually means rearranging the habits of years, which, though they may be destructive, are known and comfortable to all. We should not underestimate the courage and tenacity that are required for this kind of major life change.

MELISSA'S STORY: SABOTAGE AND TRIUMPH

Over the past 4 years, Melissa Humphreys (not her real name) has managed to lose 80 pounds and keep off most of them. She's accomplished this feat through enrollment in a university-based Low Calorie

Diet. For her, the keys to maintenance of her lower weight have been regular exercise, learning how to cope with supersize restaurant portions, and dealing with the emotional complications presented by family and friends.

Her family meant well, but their constant comments about her weight—dating to her childhood—were not helpful in slimming down. A roommate with a drinking problem had to drop out of her life entirely before she was ready to lose weight. One boyfriend with a superiority complex was less than not helpful—he was an actual hindrance.

> *By the time she left college and moved to the United States, Melissa weighed 200 to 220 pounds.*

Through it all, Melissa kept her eyes on the bottom line and today likes herself and her life better than ever before. Her story illustrates the multifaceted nature of a successful weight-loss program, in which restricting diet and boosting exercise comprise only half the battle. The other half is controlling those aspects of life that lie outside the clinic—the everyday tugs of war and hour-by-hour choices that control your fate once you leave the special foods, supplement shakes, and official scales behind for the last time.

At the time of our interview, Melissa was 32 years old. She stood 5 feet, 7 inches and weighed about 170 pounds—not svelte, exactly, but healthy. She was aiming for 150 pounds but thinking she would be satisfied with 160 as a maintenance weight. Melissa grew up in England, of "good Welsh stock," and says she as well as others in her family have always been big-boned and "chunky." Of those in her family, though, only she became seriously obese. Unfortunately, that singled her out for extra attention, comment, and speculation beginning at an early age.

"I have been overweight all my life, maybe from the age of 3 onward," she says. "By the age of 8, I was definitely bigger than everybody else. I think from the age of 3 to 8 I just got bigger and bigger. My mother and I have discussed it many times. We really don't know why this happened. I wasn't a demanding baby, and I wasn't getting fed all the time or anything like that."

By the time she left college and moved to the United States, Melissa weighed 200 to 220 pounds. "When I came here, to the American food system, where the servings are huge, and all-you-can-eat buffets are everywhere, for someone like me, who is susceptible to not knowing when to stop, I gained another 30 to 40 pounds."

She knew she should lose weight and attended a Weight Watchers meeting—once. She did not go back. "The group meetings seemed to be a little cheesy," she says. "There was a lot of cheerleading with very little substance. But that may be me, being a Brit in an American situation."

Melissa began exercising regularly and lost weight. Then she stopped exercising and gained it back. If she ever had been tempted to forget about it, though, and just accept herself as she was, a constant stream of comments from her family would have prevented that. "Families find it very difficult when someone is overweight," she says, with some sympathy in her voice. "They do want you to lose weight. But very often, the way they go about it just makes the person run away and eat more. They just want to hide from it. They know they're overweight. Everyone knows when they're overweight. Everyone knows how to lose weight. But doing it is the difficult thing."

> *Families find it very difficult when someone is overweight. They do want you to lose weight. But very often, the way they go about it just makes the person run away and eat more.*
>
> —MELISSA

Melissa learned there was a comprehensive weight-loss clinic at the university where she was employed as a computer consultant. A year before she finally enrolled, she visited the program and received an explanation of what would be involved if she chose to enroll. However, "My living situation would not have been conducive to losing weight, because I was living with someone who drank quite a bit of alcohol. Not being able to drink alcohol when you're living with someone who drinks quite a bit was going to be awkward. So finally, I moved out and was living on my own, and that's when I started the program."

At the time she first registered, 4 years ago, Melissa weighed 252 pounds. She is convinced her top weight was closer to 270. However, the moment she decided to join the program, she became conscious of what she ate and began to shed pounds. From May 1997, when she joined the program and went on a low-calorie diet with special nutritional supplements, to December 1997, when she finished that diet, Melissa lost 80 pounds.

Compared to the serious work of maintaining a weight loss in the real world, losing weight initially with the low-calorie diet is easy, Melissa says. She calls it "la-la land."

"You're in this funny land where food is totally controlled," she says. "The real advantage of it is the (near) fast. You're almost guaranteed to lose weight. You're eating somewhere between 800 and 1,400 calories a day. Some people lose 6 pounds a week. It's a great tool to lose weight quickly and in such a manner that you can keep your momentum going. In every other diet program that I've seen, you lose half a pound or a pound, and you feel like you're being deprived. It's very difficult to keep yourself going. Whereas on the supplements, your hunger goes away or is greatly reduced. You don't really have choices.

> *As compared with losing weight in the first place—especially on a medically supervised Low Calorie Diet—maintaining the weight loss is difficult, Melissa admits.*

"You have five supplements a day, and you have 4 ounces of chicken, or 4 ounces of meat, and salad and dressing. Your choice of dressings is limited as well. It's easier, because you don't have to think—should I have a candy bar? You know if you have a candy bar, you're going to be kicked out of ketosis, and you'll suddenly be hungry again. So you've got all these good reasons not to cheat."

As compared with losing weight in the first place—especially on a medically supervised Low Calorie Diet—maintaining the weight loss is difficult, Melissa admits. "The fast is easy, but it is the learning how to maintain and deal with food afterward that is the really, really hard bit," she says. "I didn't congratulate myself on losing the weight. I was proud of myself for losing the weight, but I didn't feel that I had done my job until a year later, when I had kept it off. I know it's the learning how to deal with food that helped me keep it off."

One of Melissa's secrets: "I don't have candy around. If I can't control myself with a certain food, I no longer buy it." She keeps carrots and apples around the house for quick snacks.

Another secret is always to ask for doggie bags in restaurants. Don't try to eat the whole thing. "In the U.K., doggie bags are frowned upon," says Melissa. "But then again, portion sizes are considerably smaller. Whereas here, doggie bags are encouraged. So I use that. I take things home."

Over the course of 4 years, Melissa's weight has gone up and down. She has actually gone through the fast twice. After she shed 80 pounds the first time, her weight crept up. But she knew why, and she learned how to take corrective action. "Even now when I have a stressful situation, my relationship with food changes," she says.

"When I'm feeling really bad, I don't want to eat at all. When I'm feeling bad but not terrible, I want food. I want to hide and comfort myself with food. Food is a comfort. It always has been a comfort. Our mothers fed us when we were crying. It tastes good."

Now Melissa has learned to reward herself in other ways than with food. She suggests getting a pedicure, having a massage, or going clothes shopping. After all, she needed to replace her entire wardrobe after she lost the 80 pounds.

> Melissa has learned to reward herself in other ways than with food. She suggests getting a pedicure, having a massage, or going clothes shopping. After all, she needed to replace her entire wardrobe after she lost the 80 pounds.

About 3 years after she initially went through the fast and experienced her dramatic weight loss, Melissa realized she had regained about 20 pounds. Part of it was due to a visit back home to England, where she ate too much. Part of it was due to a breakup with a boyfriend, after which she gained more weight. Part of it was due to a medication she was taking for an unrelated medical condition. "So about a month ago I started on the program again," she said. "I have lost about 15 pounds this month. On average, I lose about 3 pounds a week on the program. I am aiming to go down to 150 and planning that my real weight will end up being at 160."

There are two additional keys to Melissa's confidence: having clarified her personal life and having committed herself to regular, enjoyable exercise.

At the beginning of her initial fast, Melissa recalls, she had a boyfriend who, in retrospect, liked her just the way she was—because he could feel superior to her. The psychologist in her weight program asks participants at the beginning to think about who will try to sabotage their weight loss. Almost invariably, it is the people closest to them, "because in many ways, people don't like change. It upsets the balance," Melissa explains.

> *There are two additional keys to Melissa's confidence: having clarified her personal life and having committed herself to regular, enjoyable exercise.*

In this case, Melissa's boyfriend simply stopped talking to her when she started the fast. They had been very close, spending every weekend together. But suddenly, "he didn't talk to me for 3 or 4 months. He said later that he was trying to make me stand on my own two feet. But I think he found it very threatening that I was trying to do something about a major problem in my life that didn't involve him. I was no longer doing things the way he wanted them done." After she lost the weight, their relationship ended.

"Before I lost the weight, it was sort of me wanting a relationship with him. After I lost the weight, he wanted a relationship with me. But after going through his not talking with me for a couple of months, and after having other people start reminding me that I am a good person, and having other men make comments that I was attractive, I was not interested in him. And I think that was what he was scared of. I was always there, always available. If he decided to look at me, I was available. And suddenly, I wasn't anymore."

Nor is her experience unique, Melissa says. For years, she has been attending the weekly support group maintained by the weight-loss program, which she finds invaluable. Another woman in her group had similar problems with her partner. "They're superior. They're better," says Melissa, describing such partners. "They can just squeeze you in various ways, because you've got the weight problem. If your self-confidence is low already, they chip at it in other places to make it lower. What it's showing is someone who does not have much confidence in themselves. It's a way of making them feel better about themselves, like a bully."

Also transformed was Melissa's relationship with her family, back home in England. "I am still the biggest in my family, but only by a size or maybe two sizes. But by far, I am the most active in my family. I exercise far more than anyone else in my family. They still talk about my weight, which is okay, but in some ways I wish it would no longer be an issue that would be discussed. I never talk about their weight. When I go home now, I go out for walks with my mother, or we go out and do things that are much more active. They're more fun to do now, whereas before, they were a chore."

That point, in itself, illustrates the new mobility in Melissa's life. She is much more active and has much more self-confidence.

"There is a huge amount of difference," she says. "I refer to the 'old me' and the 'new me.' The physical change facilitated a mental change. I can run up a flight of stairs without worrying about it. I can sit in airplane seats without having to stretch the safety belt around me. I lost 10 inches from my waist when I lost 80 pounds. I went from a size 26 to a size 14. My shoes went down a size as well. And it was lovely going to a regular-size store and not having to go to the large-size stores."

> *Melissa calls herself a "black-and-white person" who follows instructions to the letter. She believes she will continue to comply with the terms of her new lifestyle. But she also acknowledges that vigilance will be required for the rest of her life.*

As she looks to the future, Melissa is confident that she will always stay close to her goal weight. She has become fanatical about badminton—not the sedate picnic sport, but the serious competitive version played in the Olympics, with players smashing the shuttle at each other at speeds of more than 100 miles per hour. "It's a workout," she laughs.

As a computer specialist, Melissa calls herself a "black-and-white person" who follows instructions to the letter. She believes she will continue to comply with the terms of her new lifestyle. But she also acknowledges that vigilance will be required for the rest of her life.

"If I don't keep it consciously in my mind, being aware of it all the time, I can slip down that slide again," she says. "It's something I am going to have to be aware of always. If I fall off the track, I just need to go to the right places to get help."

SOCIETY'S TREATMENT OF THE OBESE

At the beginning of the 21st century, one unfortunate fact of life has not changed for many obese people. Despite the fact that both their absolute number and their proportion in the population continue to grow year by year, they are still the targets of pity, condescension, and doubt. Study after study has documented the fact that obese people are stereotyped as lazy and weak and that they face an uphill climb to reach a level playing field in many arenas of life—the classroom, the workplace, and even such intimate aspects of daily life as their prospects for marriage.

For those of us who have spent years working with obese people and admiring their struggle and determination in the face of daunting challenges, these are particularly troubling examples of prejudice. Unfortunately, they are widespread and unthinking forms of criticism, which begin for many overweight people when they are still children.

Our hope must be that the messages contained in books such as this—that obesity is a medical condition with tangled genetic, biochemical, social, cultural, and behavioral roots—will begin to change perceptions of the obese. All of society has a stake in understanding and rolling back the tide of obesity, not because it is a personal failing, but because it often has serious health and quality-of-life consequences for the individual. Fortunately, some signs indicate that a medical understanding of obesity is beginning to penetrate the public consciousness and to change the ways in which the obese are treated in the law and in our economy.

Obesity and Taxes

In 2000, the American Obesity Association (AOA), representing a variety of groups with interests in the issue (including Jenny Craig and Weight Watchers, among others), won important concessions from the Internal Revenue Service (IRS) when the IRS agreed, for the first time, to allow taxpayers to deduct the cost of weight-loss measures that are prescribed by their doctor for the treatment of disease. (See sidebar, Tax Deduction for the Obese.) The AOA argued successfully that obesity should be considered as a medical condition whose successful treatment in turn prevents the development of a number of diseases.[19]

"The new IRS policy will provide much needed assistance to individuals and families faced with devastating medical bills incurred from treating conditions that can be alleviated with weight loss," said AOA executive director Morgan Downey, in announcing the new policy. In an interview, he explained that medical deductions will be difficult to claim for many taxpayers because of the high threshold that must be reached. Taxpayers must be able to claim 7.5 percent of their adjusted gross income as medical expenses to qualify for the deduction. But the new IRS policy also makes it possible for people to use pretax dollars from their Flexible Savings Accounts or Medical Savings Accounts at

> *The new IRS policy also makes it possible for people to use pretax dollars from their Flexible Savings Accounts or Medical Savings Accounts to pay for weight-loss treatments.*

work to pay for weight-loss treatments. This change will allow many more people to benefit from the new guideline.

Interestingly, the new policy does not allow deductions for weight-loss treatments simply to maintain good health, even if they are prescribed by a doctor. Nor does it define *overweight* or *obesity*. Defending the medical necessity of a weight-loss program will be up to the taxpayer and his or her accountant, subject, of course, to audit review by the IRS. The AOA suggests making a note for your files or, better yet, obtaining a letter from your doctor containing the instruction to lose weight for medical reasons.

Tax Deduction for the Obese: What's Allowable, What's Not

The new interpretation (as of December 2000) contained in IRS Publication 502 says, "You cannot include the cost of a weight-loss program in medical expenses [for deduction] if the purpose of the weight control is to maintain your general good health. But you can include the cost of a weight-loss program undertaken at a physician's direction to treat an existing disease (such as heart disease)."

Having won this important point with the IRS, the American Obesity Association faces larger battles ahead with Medicare, Medicaid, and private insurers to cover the costs of the entire range of medical treatments for obesity. In general, AOA executive director Morgan Downey says, private health insurance companies seem more inclined to pay for bariatric surgery than for drug treatment or behavioral counseling—principally because studies have been able to document good, long-term outcomes for bariatric surgery. "The surgeons have long waiting lines for their services and have been getting more and more insurers to cover the procedure," he says.

Allowable

According to the AOA's interpretation, potentially allowable expenses would include:

If you are interested in exploring this deduction, consult your own accountant or tax adviser. You may find, depending on your personal situation, that your pocketbook has new grounds for hope.

OBESITY IN CHILDREN AND TEENS

In the 1970s, author Paul Ehrlich publicized the concept of the "Population Bomb." His thesis was that the world's rapidly growing population would outstrip the Earth's ecological capacity, leading to catastrophe for the human race.

- Bariatric surgery
- Prescription (FDA-approved) anti-obesity drugs
- Weight-reduction programs directed by a doctor or hospital
- Behavioral counseling
- Professional services of physicians, dietitians, or nutritionists
- Commercial programs for weight loss and maintenance[20]

Not Allowable
The FDA's new ruling will *not* allow deductions for:

- Cosmetic surgery, including liposuction
- Exercise equipment
- Health club dues
- Low-fat foods
- Nonprescription drugs and medicines
- Nutritional supplements, including vitamins, herbal supplements, or natural medicines, "unless you can only obtain them legally with a physician's prescription"[21]

These days, not much is heard about that particular time bomb (though some may still think it an apt metaphor). But in another, almost equally alarming sense, our population is indeed exploding. The waistlines of the youngest people in our society are growing rapidly. And a form of medical catastrophe may be in the offing.

In the past decade, the percentage of America's children and teens who are overweight or obese has nearly doubled. In the past 20 years, the percentage has nearly *tripled*. Alarmed doctors are warning that the first early warning signs of obesity—in the form of type 2 diabetes in very young people—are already being seen, decades earlier in the life span than has been the case with past generations. By the time these obese youngsters are in their 20s and 30s, many doctors warn, the damage will be done; it will be too late.

> Honesty about the situation we face may help some parents take an unvarnished look at their own children and begin to make changes in their family diet and lifestyle while there is still time to do so.

This is not a pretty picture. Signs of hope are few. This is one case in which it appears that the night will get darker, from a public health standpoint, before the first light of dawn will be seen. But if nothing else, honesty about the situation we face may help some parents take an unvarnished look at their own children and begin to make changes in their family diet and lifestyle while there is still time to do so. It is also possible that sufficiently alarmed and insistent parents' groups may help to trigger changes in schools, in fast-food marketing, and in our sedentary culture that will save future generations of kids from premature illness and debility related to obesity.

What Are the Facts?

If it seems like you see more children who are obviously rotund when you go to the mall or the grocery store, statistics say you're right. The percentage of overweight and obese children in America has nearly doubled in the past 10 years. And there is no sign that the trend is slowing or reversing. The situation is so alarming that the surgeon general of the United States devoted a special section to children and teens in his "call to action" to prevent obesity in late 2001. The warning from Dr. David Satcher was similar in urgency to previous surgeons general advisories about the dangers of cigarette smoking or unprotected sex in the light of AIDS.[22] Many doctors believe that from a medical standpoint, obesity—especially in the very young—is nearly a comparable threat to the health of Americans.

The most recent authoritative study was done by two researchers from the University of Michigan and the New Jersey College of Medicine and Dentistry, Drs. Richard Strauss and Harold Pollack. Writing in the *Journal of the American Medical Association*, they reported that overweight increased by 120 percent (that is, more than doubled) in 4- to 12-year-old African American and Hispanic children from 1986 to 1998. During this period, overweight increased by about 50 percent among white children. Based on a study of 8,720 children enrolled in the National Longitudinal Study of Youth, more than 21 percent of African American children, more than 21 percent of Hispanic children, and more than 12 percent of non-Hispanic whites are overweight, they said. And overweight children tracked in the study are heavier today than they were 15 years ago, the researchers added. Concluding that "urgency is warranted in responding to this epidemic," they also acknowledged there are no simple answers to the problem, with many causes common to adults as well as to children in our society.[23] In other words, our children are unlikely to change unless the weight problem is addressed in adults as well.

> *Our children are unlikely to change unless the weight problem is addressed in adults as well.*

At the same time, U.S. Surgeon General David Satcher estimates that 14 percent of adolescents, ages 12 to 19, are overweight, a percentage that has nearly tripled in the past 20 years.[24]

How Do You Measure Obesity in a Child?

Recall that in chapter 2, we introduced the concept of Body Mass Index (BMI); gave several different ways of calculating it for any given person; and explained that a person with a BMI greater than or equal to 25 is considered overweight, while a BMI greater than or equal to 30 is considered obese.

Not surprising, perhaps, it is not quite this simple for children and adolescents. Although the BMI is calculated in the same way as for adults (see chapter 2), its meaning and interpretation are different. From infancy through adolescence, youngsters go through predictable patterns of weight gain and growth, making simple arithmetic formulas misleading. Doctors have developed the concept of BMI-for-age—or BMI with respect to others in their peer group—to gauge overweight in children and teens. Thus, from ages 2 to 20, *underweight* is defined as a BMI-for-age of less than the 5th percentile. In other words, if 95 percent of other children of the same age have a greater BMI, a child is considered underweight. A BMI-for-age greater than or equal to the 85th percentile is defined as *at risk for overweight*. So, if only 15 percent of other children that age have a greater BMI, a child is at risk. Having a BMI-for-age greater than or equal to the 95th percentile is defined as *overweight*.[25]

Further complicating the matter, the BMI-for-age formulas for boys and girls are different. This is certainly one case in which a picture (or, more precisely, a chart) is worth a thousand words (see figures 7.1 and 7.2).

What Causes Childhood Obesity?

All parents know the sometimes flattering, sometimes uncomfortable sensation of seeing themselves reflected, for good and ill, in the attitudes and behavior of their children. So it is with the problem of overweight in our youngsters. They're growing up to be just like us. In the main, the reasons for their overweight problems are the same as ours: bad diets, including too much fast food and snack food, and not enough physical activity.

To a greater degree than ever before, children today have been weaned on the electronic baby-sitter, the television. According to the

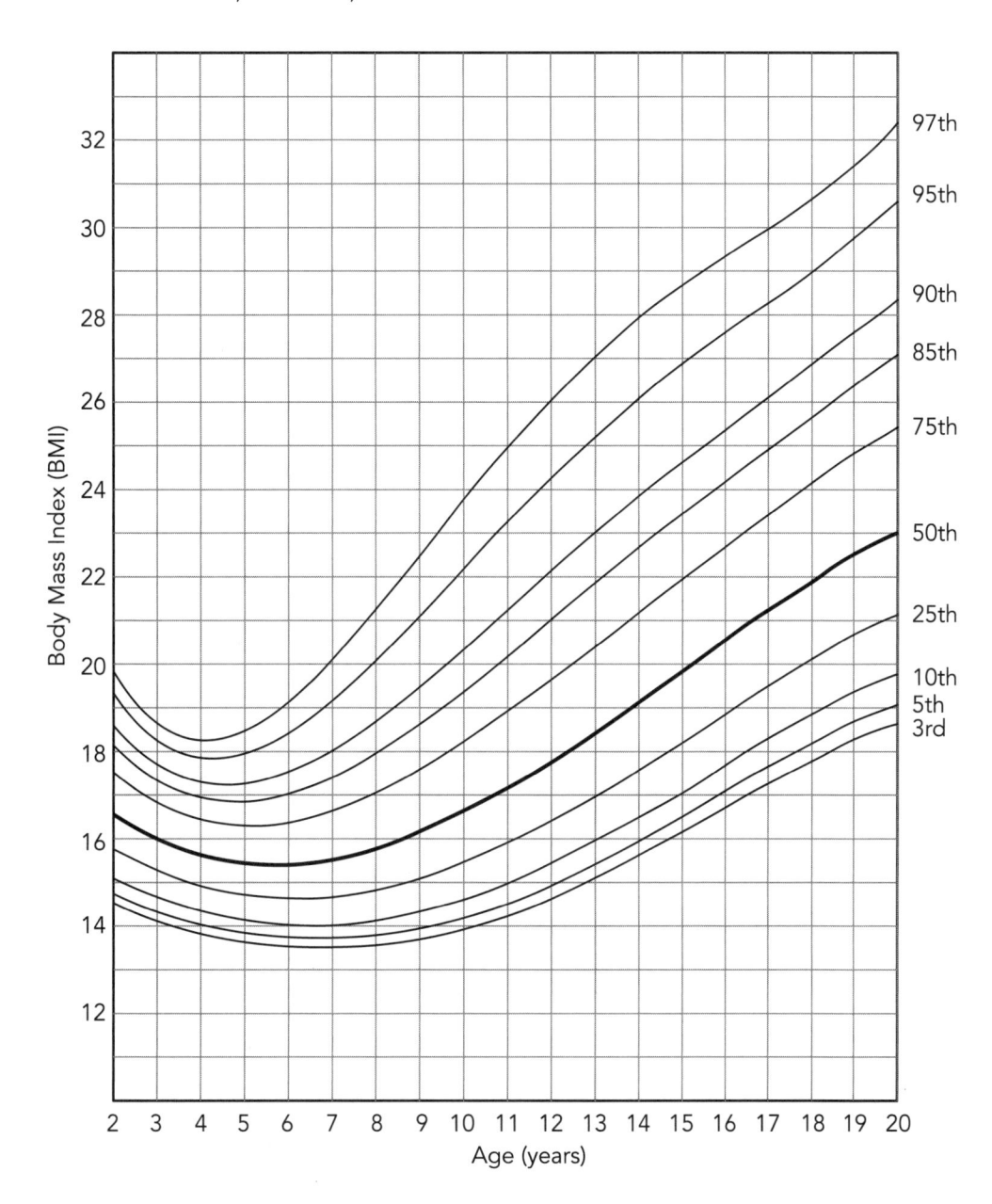

Figure 7.1—*Body Mass Index-for-Age Percentiles for Boys (2–20 Years)*

Source: Developed by the National Center for Health Statistics with the National Center for Chronic Disease Prevention and Health Promotion, 2000.

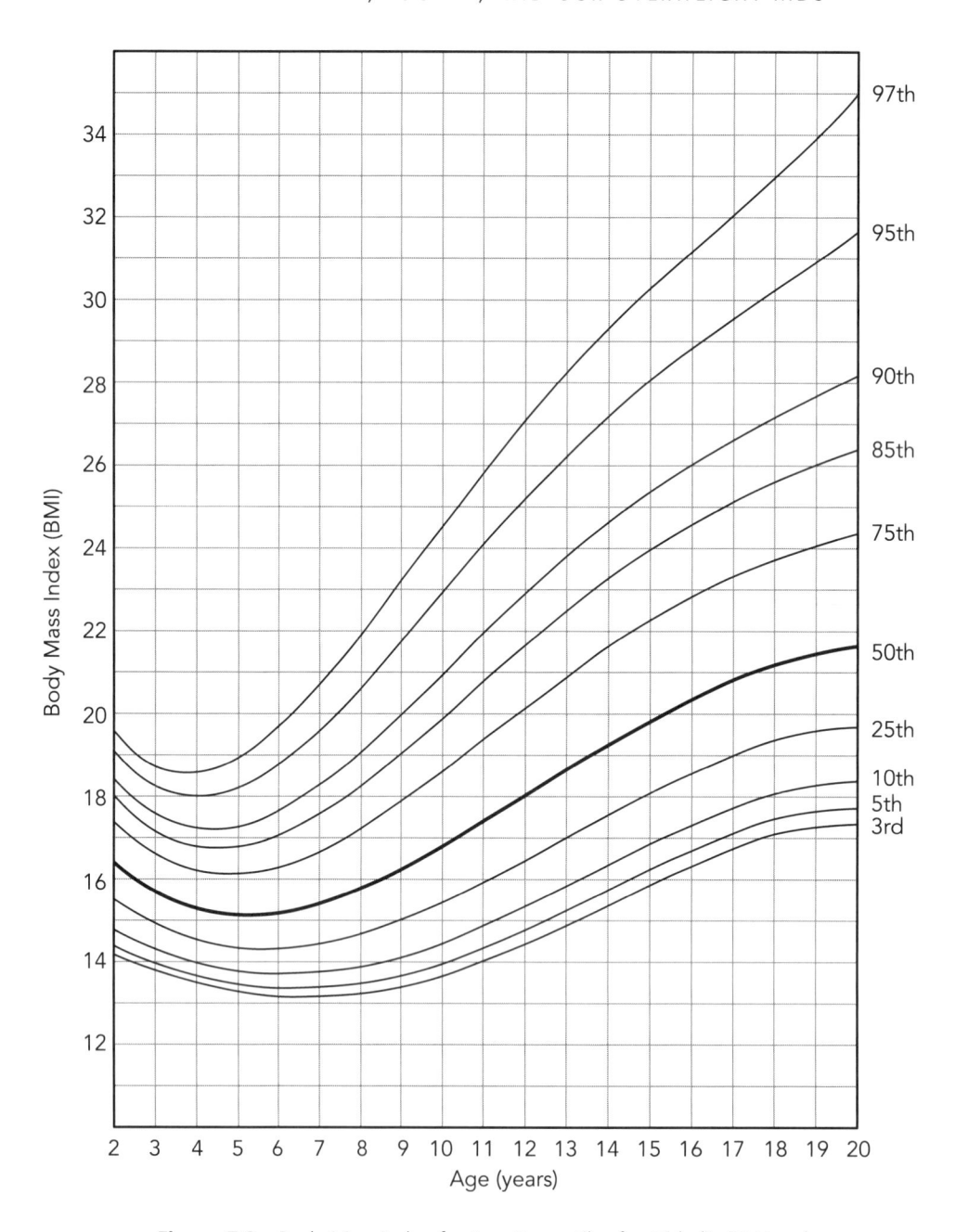

Figure 7.2—*Body Mass Index-for-Age Percentiles for Girls (2–20 Years)*

Source: Developed by the National Center for Health Statistics with the National Center for Chronic Disease Prevention and Health Promotion, 2000.

surgeon general's report, more than 40 percent of American teens watch more than 2 hours of TV a day. In addition, they are the first generation to devote substantial amounts of recreational time to playing video games and surfing the Web on their personal computers. Children and teens spend fewer hours each day in outdoor activities and exercise. According to the AOA, today only one-quarter of the nation's high school students receive daily physical education.[26] The AOA says daily PE classes have declined by 30 percent in the past decade, often as schools try to cram in more classroom time so their students perform better on standardized tests.

Other advocacy groups criticize the widespread availability of snack and soda machines in schools. Studies have shown that children who drink as little as one soda or sweetened drink a day are more likely than those who do not to gain extra weight over time.[27]

In addition to these general considerations, the following key stages of development seem to be of critical importance in determining whether children become obese.

In the womb. Babies born to mothers who have diabetes, whether that diabetes is type 1, type 2, or gestation induced, tend to be fatter at birth. Although these babies tend to lose their excess weight by 1 year of age, they also tend to become heavier than their peers several years later in childhood.

At the age of 4 to 5. Children go through a phase known as "adiposity rebound." Their BMI reaches its lowest point and then begins to climb again as their bodies prepare for their growth spurt in adolescence. Children who "rebound" from this dip earlier than others are more prone to obesity.

Adolescence. Especially in girls, obesity in adolescence is predictive of obesity in later life. Some studies have shown that about 30 percent of obese women were obese as teens, while the same was true of only 10 percent of obese men.[28]

What Are the Consequences of Childhood Obesity?

Obesity in childhood and adolescence frequently carries over into adult life, as noted earlier. It carries a risk of early development of type 2 diabetes and cardiovascular disease. "Type 2 diabetes is primarily related to people being overweight," says Dr. Robert Berkowitz, an associate professor at the University of Pennsylvania School of Medicine. "I never saw type 2 diabetes in children 20 years ago, and now the National Institutes of Health is awarding grants to study the phenomenon."[29]

Doctors who specialize in treating diabetes and who are aware of its potentially devastating long-term implications are especially alarmed.

> *Obesity in childhood and adolescence frequently carries over into adult life. It carries a risk of early development of type 2 diabetes and cardiovascular disease.*

"What used to be a disease in Grandma and Grandpa is now a disease in children and young adults," says Dr. Curtiss Cook, an Emory University endocrinologist who practices at a diabetes clinic in urban Atlanta. "We are seeing people in their 20s and 30s who already have complications. Tackling the problem of diabetes should be a national priority."

Even without the real risk of disease, obesity in childhood and the teen years exacts a cruel price in terms of social stigmatism and ostracism by other children. Oddly, some evidence shows that the social situation is getting worse rather than better, even as overweight kids are more numerous than ever. A recent study in which middle-school children were shown drawings of children who were healthy, obese, or disabled shows that expressed dislike of obese children has grown in the 40 years since the same experiment was originally done. At the same time, thin kids were rated as more likable.[30]

An additional cruelty exacted by childhood and teenage obesity is that its negative effects ripple through all dimensions of a child's life, for years to come. Even when researchers control for such variables as parents' income, parents' education, and ethnicity, obese people are at a disadvantage. Table 9, prepared by researcher William Dietz of Tufts University, summarizes the effects of obesity on young women in a national survey, as compared to normal-weight peers. Obesity was defined as having a BMI greater than the 95th percentile of women the same age in the survey.

What Can We Do About It?

In some respects, the prescriptions for overweight youngsters are precisely the same as those for their corpulent parents:

- If your child is very obese, talk to his or her doctor before starting a weight-management program.
- Make sure your child eats a balanced diet with at least five servings of fruits and vegetables a day.
- Start your child's day with a healthful breakfast.
- Serve fruits and veggies for snacks, not chips and cookies.

Table 9. Effects of Obesity in Young Women

Outcome	Adjusted Difference
Schooling	−0.3 years
Marriage	−20 percent
Household income	−$6,710
Poverty	+10 percent

Source: W. H. Dietz, "Prevalence of Obesity in Children," in *Handbook of Obesity*, ed. G. A. Bray, C. Bouchard, and W. P. T. James (New York: Dekker, 1998).

- Do not allow your child to eat while watching TV.
- Ensure that your child is physically active and does not spend much leisure time watching TV, playing video or computer games, or surfing on the Internet.

But in some important respects, the recommended goals for obese children and teens are different from those of adults:

- Your child should get 60 minutes (1 hour) of physical exercise a day, twice the 30-minute minimum recommended for adults.
- In many cases, weight reduction will not be the recommended goal for obese youngsters. Many children and teens will "grow into" their weight. A more appropriate goal may be to hold their current weight steady as their height increases. Recall our discussion of the BMI in children being somewhat variable as they pass through their developmental stages. Again, your family doctor or child's pediatrician will likely be in the best position to advise you.[31]

A final note: No matter how overweight a child may be, remember that he or she is likely getting a bountiful measure of teasing and negative comments from schoolmates. Children need our loving, intelligent support, not constant nagging and criticism. If anything, a negative approach will only backfire and may further impair self-esteem. Your best chance of reversing childhood obesity is to change the diet and behavior of your entire family—including yourself. The reason for making these behavior and diet changes must be understood and communicated to your child as being good for health and fun, not in any way as a punishment or as confirmation of the false and unfair societal prejudice that obesity is a personal failing. The family that walks and plays together, slims down and lives longer together.

> *The family that walks and plays together, slims down and lives longer together.*

CHAPTER 8

On the Horizon

THE 21ST CENTURY will see a whole range of artillery brought to bear against the epidemic of obesity. Medical science will declare war with all of the new findings and products of genetic medicine. It is not impossible to imagine that scores of new drugs, hormones, and neurotransmitters will be tailored to the genetic profile of each obese person. In this way, the treatment of obesity will become as sophisticated as that of cancer therapy, which is already moving in this direction.

However, as thousands of disappointed biotech investors can attest, the future of molecular medicine has been just around the corner for a long time now. We may safely predict that the glories of genetically customized obesity treatment are still, at best, a decade or two away. This view is particularly valid given the painful history of anti-obesity drugs, which frequently have unforeseen side effects precisely to the extent that they are effective in reducing weight—such as fen-phen and amphetamines. New drugs will be developed; indeed, we will review some promising candidates later in this chapter. But they will take longer to come on line than many might wish.

In the meantime, new drugs will not exhaust the full spectrum of what medicine will have to offer. Other prospects include the following:

- New medical devices to help reduce appetite, especially in the morbidly obese—possibly including inflatable gastric balloons and electrical implants.
- The development of more synthetic nonfattening dietary ingredients such as olestra.

At the same time, many doctors will continue to recommend bariatric surgery for the morbidly obese. Others, more conservative in their approach, will take advantage of a growing body of insights into how successful dieters have been able to lose substantial amounts of weight and to keep it off.

But with 61 percent of American adults—three out of every five—now considered overweight or obese, public health initiatives will be as important as medical advances in treating obesity, as they are for battling other medical conditions. After many decades of intense work, doctors still cannot treat lung cancer or emphysema, for example, as effectively as they can prevent their occurrence by reducing smoking. Therefore, as the tide of obesity continues to advance, public health approaches will become ever more important. It will be a long time—if ever—before a surgeon's general warning is slapped on the sides of ice cream containers or bags of potato chips. But it may not be so long before you become aware of a growing volume—and urgency—of medical warnings about the need to be slim and trim. You will also note an increasing emphasis on changes that must occur at the societal level—ranging from better, safer access to walking and biking trails, to greater concern about the exercise and dietary habits of schoolchildren.

> As the tide of obesity continues to advance, public health approaches will become ever more important.

Increasingly, the government (especially Medicare), corporations, and insurers will recognize that obesity is too serious a health condition, and too costly in terms of both the associated disease burden and the nation's hospital bills, to shrug off. This awareness will dominate public discussion in the years ahead.

MEDICAL ADVANCES

Let's take a look now at some of the contributions medical science is making in helping overcome obesity, including a sample of the latest drug treatments, medical devices, food supplements, and behavioral research.

Drug Treatment

In chapter 1, we discussed the discovery of the hormone leptin, which is produced by adipose tissue (the body's fat stores) and is a crucial part of the feedback mechanism between brain and body that regulates appetite and eating. Leptin appears to be involved in a complex array of biochemical signals and effects, and it may also increase the body's metabolic rate, specifically promoting the metabolism of fat.[1] From the mid-1990s on, hundreds of researchers have trained their sights on leptin and on the receptors in the brain that detect its presence in the body. In both animal models and humans, the failure to produce leptin leads to obesity. Given this elementary fact, many researchers have believed leptin would be the basis of the first highly effective, safe drug to fight obesity. And it still may—but progress has been slower than first expected when Amgen paid $20 million in 1995 to license the rights to the leptin gene from Rockefeller University.

> *Many researchers have believed leptin would be the basis of the first highly effective, safe drug to fight obesity. And it still may—but progress has been slower than first expected.*

For one thing, researchers have learned there is no simple correlation between the level of leptin in the blood and someone's degree of obesity. That is, the presence of leptin does not appear automatically to register the presence of sufficient fat reserves and shut down an obese person's hypothalamus-triggered appetite. According to National Institutes of Health researchers Jack Yanovski and Susan Yanovski, "The vast majority of obese individuals appear to have normal genetic sequences for leptin and its receptor, and have high levels of leptin in proportion to their body fat stores."[2]

Nevertheless, leptin clearly is a key ingredient in the appetite–energy–obesity equation, and work continues on development of a commercially viable drug form. In 1999, Amgen sponsored a trial of leptin in 127 people at four university weight loss clinics and two contract laboratories. The study showed that daily injections of leptin (it must be injected since it is a small peptide molecule that would be inactivated by digestive enzymes if taken orally) produced weight loss that varied directly with the amount of the dose—the more leptin administered, the greater the weight loss.[3] Some data suggested that resistance to the effects of leptin increases as people grow more obese. No clinically significant side effects were noted other than irritation at the injection site and headache. Understandably, the researchers concluded that further study is warranted. In fact, Amgen is currently involved in phase 2 clinical trials of a second-generation recombinant (artificially produced) form of leptin for the treatment of obesity.

> *Obese people may develop resistance to the slimming effects of leptin, whether it is naturally generated in their own bodies or administered as a drug.*

However, if taking a daily shot of leptin to treat obesity sounds about as appealing as injecting insulin to control diabetes, your reaction is probably the same as that of many individuals. And oddly, the comparison may be more than skin-deep here. Just as leptin is produced by fatty tissue, so insulin is produced in greater and greater quantities as individuals grow more obese—but by the pancreas rather than the body's fat stores. You may recall that this phenomenon leads to growing insulin intolerance (insulin resistance), which is a precursor to the development of type 2 diabetes. Similarly, obese people may develop resistance to the slimming effects of leptin, whether it is naturally generated in their own bodies or administered as a drug.

An article in the *Journal of the American Medical Association* notes that leptin and insulin "share many properties as adiposity signals . . .

the secretion of both hormones is influenced by the overall amount of fat stores as well as by short-term changes in energy balance. Moreover, insulin receptors are located in the same key hypothalamic areas as leptin receptors."[4] An additional factor in explaining why obese individuals may be leptin-resistant is the possibility that the physiological signal is ignored. In other words, even in the presence of a hormonal signal that a person is satiated, that person may quite possibly eat anyway.

The relationship among leptin, insulin, obesity, and diabetes will continue to be one of the most complex, sometimes contradictory, and intensely studied areas in medicine. Stay tuned for interesting developments.

Exciting as the leptin research is, it does not exhaust the fertile ground for new drug development. Some of the most promising new anti-obesity candidates have raised considerable interest by taking advantage of different pathways to lessen appetite or inhibit the digestion of dietary fats. Researchers Jack Yanovski and Susan Yanovski have described a number of different systems at the molecular level that might become targets for anti-obesity treatments. They include several neurotransmitters that affect appetite and eating (neuropeptide Y, pro-opiomelanocortin, melanocyte stimulating hormone, the endorphins, and the enkephalins); a gene mutation that may literally increase the number of fat cells in the body; and a group of proteins that may be capable of diverting excess energy into heat rather than having it stored within the cell.

> Some of the most promising new anti-obesity candidates have raised considerable interest by taking advantage of different pathways to lessen appetite or inhibit the digestion of dietary fats.

Researchers have also observed a substantial difference between people in terms of their tendency to burn energy through "nonresting" activities. These would include the propensity to "fidget," maintaining one's posture, and other subtle activities of daily living that do not qualify as exercise but, nevertheless, can result in a person's expending energy rather than being stuck with excess calories that have nowhere to go other than storage as fat. A recent study of how various people responded to a program of intentional overfeeding "leads to the intriguing possibility that we might decrease the prevalence of obesity by instructing people to fidget more," write Yanovski and Yanovski.[5]

Meanwhile, scarcely a month goes by without news of some new candidate for anti-obesity drug development. Here are three recent examples.

C75. In June 2000, a group of scientists from Johns Hopkins University published a paper in *Science*, saying they had produced a compound called C75 that apparently interferes with the production of neuropeptide Y in mice. Without neuropeptide Y, obese mice experienced a sharp drop in appetite and lost weight rapidly. The effects of C75, belonging to a group of organic molecules called the butyrolactones, seemed to wear off once injections were stopped and mice resumed normal feeding, with no apparent toxic effects. Continuing their research into the possible anti-obesity drug properties of C75, the same scientists, in December 2001, published a study of C75 in lean and genetically obese mice that furthers our understanding of how the compound works. C75-treated mice seem to ignore hunger signals because the drug blocks fatty acid synthase, an enzyme in the body that is needed to break down malonyl CoA, a regulator of the levels of various brain chemicals like neuropeptide Y that affect appetite. Thus, the C75-treated mice do not adjust the levels of the appetite-affecting neurochemicals in their brains appropriately in response to fasting, so they do not get hungry. What is unknown is whether the appetite-suppressing effect will be lasting with continued treatment, or whether another part of the neuroendocrine system of checks and balances will take over and work around the effect of the C75.[6]

ACC2 blocker. In a March 2001 article in *Science*, researchers from the Baylor College of Medicine reported that blocking the production of an enzyme called ACC2 in genetically engineered mice interfered with the normal formation of fatty acids. Instead, the mitochondria (subcellular organelles sometimes described as the cell's powerhouse) in these mice burned fat continuously, allowing them to eat up to 40 percent more than normal mice while still weighing 10 to 15 percent less.[7]

Axokine. Meanwhile, the Regeneron company continues to develop a potential anti-obesity drug called axokine. Rather like the Hopkins compound, C75, that was discovered during cancer research, axokine was originally tested as a possible treatment for amylotrophic lateral sclerosis (ALS, or Lou Gehrig's disease). However, loss of appetite and weight loss turned out to be side effects. Subsequent studies in mice showed that axokine could produce a weight loss of up to 30 percent in 3 weeks without toxic side effects. The company believes that axokine, which has certain similarities to leptin but works on different receptors, may be effective in obese people who are leptin-resistant. It plans to conduct clinical trials in obese people and in people with type 2 diabetes.[8]

As we enter a new century, with the prospect of new drug treatments from these and many other lines of research, some fundamental questions about the entire enterprise remain unanswered. They are well summarized in a recent article in the *Journal of the American Medical Association* by researcher David Williamson. Briefly paraphrased, these questions are as follows:

- Can taking weight loss drugs bring about clinically significant improvements in people if they do not also make changes in their lifestyle at the same time?
- Even assuming that weight loss drugs work to some modest degree, will that result succeed in improving the quality of life that is important to people? That is, will drugs alone result in fewer heart attacks, strokes, deaths, and other adverse outcomes?

- Since there is generally a high dropout rate even in "successful" studies of weight loss drugs, will these drugs ever prove to be worthwhile for more than a minority of obese people?
- Finally, are we spending too much time and money on treating obesity rather than trying to prevent it in the population at large?

"It is hard to believe that any approach to primary prevention or to treatment of obesity will be successful at the population level without fundamental changes in cultural perceptions and expectations regarding physical activity and dietary intake," writes Williamson.[9]

Medical Devices

New drugs do not exhaust the range of possible innovative treatments for obesity. Other researchers are working on medical devices that may have a role to play as well.

BioEnterics Corporation, the company that makes the adjustable laparoscopic band discussed in chapter 5, is developing another device—an inflatable balloon that is placed in the stomach and filled with saline solution to create a feeling of fullness. According to the company, the BIB (BioEnterics Intragastric Balloon) system would be used together with a dietary and behavioral change program to produce and maintain weight loss. The system is not approved in the United States, but the company says it plans to apply to the U.S. Food and Drug Administration to begin testing the BIB as an investigational device.[10]

A second device currently under study in the United States and abroad by a company called Transneuronix is an implantable gastric stimulator, which delivers a mild electrical current to the wall of the stomach.[11] Early studies showed that pigs treated with the gastric stimulator

> BioEnterics Corporation, the company that makes the adjustable laparoscopic band, is developing another device—an inflatable balloon that is placed in the stomach and filled with saline solution to create a feeling of fullness.

experienced a reduction in feeding, followed by weight loss.[12] Research has continued, with about 200 people currently enrolled in clinical trials, the company says. Possible approval of the device and its commercial availability are still several years away, at minimum.

Food Supplements

An area that holds promise for weight control, though it has sometimes been controversial, is the concept of using nondigestible or calorie-free fat or sugar substitutes as part of the diet.

While "fat-free" or "diet" products are by no means a new idea, with lowfat, no-fat, or sugar-free versions of just about every prepared food on supermarket shelves, these products' impact on weight control remains in some doubt. Their effect is questioned, at least in part, because many people feel that they can indulge in greater quantities of such foods than their "full-fat" or "regular" versions or eat more of something else. The upshot is that they wind up not saving any of the reduced calories.

This concept is called *caloric compensation*—specifically, whether some or all of the saved calories from a reduced-calorie food are compensated for by other calories. Caloric compensation is a critically important factor in whether just about any dietary change is effective in causing weight loss.

> *The evidence is mixed, but most people do seem not to compensate fully for reduced-calorie foods and hence should be able to get some benefit from choosing these kinds of foods.*

The evidence is mixed, but most people do seem not to compensate fully for reduced-calorie foods and hence should be able to get some benefit from choosing these kinds of foods. Very interestingly, studies have shown that the calories saved by eating foods containing olestra, a nonabsorbed fat substitute, are largely not compensated for, especially when people who would normally be very restrained in their eating are not aware that they are eating a fat-free product. (Unfortunately, under normal circumstances, we are quite aware that we have chosen a reduced-calorie food. Perhaps we should learn simply to use such foods and not think about the fact that they are lower calorie!)

A related concept is that of the "energy density" of foods. High-energy-density foods pack a lot of calories and usually fat into a small volume (for example, cheese and whipped cream), while low-energy-

---

Olestra: Science at the Table

Several scientifically engineered food products are available today, and others are under development. One that has achieved some notoriety is olestra, a nonabsorbable, and thus calorie-free, fat substitute approved by the FDA for use in certain snack foods such as potato chips. It is composed of sucrose (table sugar) bonded to fatty acids. This makes olestra a compound that is not broken down by the body's digestive enzymes, so it passes through the gastrointestinal (GI) tract unchanged, appearing in the stool as an oily film. Some people have felt that they experienced diarrhea or flatulence from consuming olestra.

While this effect has been material for both jokes and complaints, careful studies indicate that olestra taken in normal quantities does not affect the GI tract much differently than when a person eats full-fat potato chips. Also of concern was the fact that fat-soluble vitamins can be lost when using olestra because they can be passed out of the GI tract along with the olestra. This effect is overcome by fortifying olestra-containing foods with extra vitamins.

While olestra (which also can appear under its commercial name, Olean, in ingredient lists) is not widely used, it is available in most supermarkets. It holds value for those of us who enjoy high-fat salty snacks and find not eating such foods unacceptable or difficult.

density foods are usually fat-free and high in water and/or fiber content (for example, most fruits, vegetables, and whole-grain starches). Dr. Barbara Rolls of Pennsylvania State University has done much research to show that we do not fully compensate when low-energy-density foods are substituted for ones with high energy density. Think of how much less filling a moderate-sized lump of cheese, at 500 calories, would be compared to 500 calories of salad greens—a full plate of very large proportions!)

While not a high-tech concept, emphasizing foods with low energy density is likely to be a winner in the future of weight control. In addition to the low-energy-density fruits and vegetables that occur naturally, food scientists are engineering other such foods and food substitutes, of which the fat substitute olestra is a leading example (see sidebar, "Olestra: Science at the Table"). Other fat substitutes are based on proteins and other foods, and thus have calories, though fewer calories than fats.

Could a Virus Cause Obesity?

Some researchers have begun working on a startling possibility: that some (or perhaps many) cases of human obesity may be due in part to otherwise unrecognized infectious disease. This would be an ironic outcome. As we have repeatedly said in this book, obesity is a disease of lifestyle caused by a multitude of factors, most prominently the mismatch between our genetic heritage and our current environment of abundant, energy-dense food and lack of physical activity. However, this does not negate the fact that a minority of cases of obesity are due to underlying medical conditions. The question is whether viral infection could be among them.

In a recent overview, researcher Richard Atkinson of the University of Wisconsin calls the possible viral connection an "ominous" possibility that urgently needs more research. He cites animal studies showing that canine distemper virus (similar to human measles) causes obesity in mice and that chickens have become obese when infected by an adenovirus. Just to show how tangled this tale could become, while these chickens became fatter, they also developed lower levels of cholesterol and triglycerides.[13]

In 2000, researchers from Wayne State University extended these lines of animal research by showing for the first time that a human adenovirus (Ad-36) could produce obesity in both chickens and mice. They found that DNA from the virus could be detected in the fat, but not in the muscles of these animals for up to 4 months following their infection. The researchers concluded that the possible role of viral infections to human obesity deserves further consideration.[14]

> *A previous unsuspected germ theory has a recent precedent in medicine. Doctors had believed prior to the late 1980s that most ulcers were caused by stress.*

At present, most doctors would say this evidence suggests a possibility rather than proof of a connection, but that is not to dismiss the idea out of hand. A previous unsuspected germ theory has a recent precedent in medicine. In the late 1980s, a young Australian doctor named Barry Marshall turned upside down the prevailing ideas about the cause of stomach ulcers. Doctors had believed prior to then that most ulcers were caused by stress. By swallowing a solution of *Helicobacter pylori*, an extremely common bacterium, previously not known to cause disease, Marshall gave himself an ulcer—which he then cured by taking antibiotics. Since then, the standard therapy for ulcers has changed completely.

Given the fact that obesity is a more complex condition than ulcers, it is very unlikely that any single germ or virus will be recognized as the culprit. But at this writing, the possibility remains alive that some viruses, in some people, could take their place in the increasingly complex jigsaw puzzle that researchers are trying to assemble.

Internet-Based Weight Programs

If the "gold standard" of weight-loss programs is the structured, weekly, face-to-face meeting of a patient with a health-care professional, it is nevertheless true that many people who could benefit from such meetings find them inconvenient and uncomfortable. For years, therapists have looked for effective alternatives. According to researchers from Brown Medical School and Virginia Tech, a well-structured program on the World Wide Web can produce moderate weight loss for some people. The researchers report in the *Journal of the American Medical Association* that a group of people who received regular Web-based behavior therapy lost an average of 10 pounds at 6 months, compared with an average loss of 3.5 pounds among a group that received only education from the same Web site.

Both groups received initial training and education in weight loss and in using the Web site, which was created by a hospital for this purpose. They got the same advice about a restricted diet to follow and minimum exercise goals. Both groups were urged to use the Web site to monitor their progress. However, the behavior therapy group also was asked to fill out an electronic diary on a weekly basis. This group also received a weekly e-mail from a therapist with general advice and personal feedback. In addition, they could use an electronic bulletin board to exchange views and experiences with fellow participants.

> According to researchers from Brown Medical School and Virginia Tech, a well-structured program on the World Wide Web can produce moderate weight loss for some people.

The latter group, perhaps not surprisingly, achieved greater weight loss and a greater reduction in their waist sizes. The researchers conclude that the weight loss was comparable to that found in a commercial weight loss program, but not as good as that usually reported in behavior therapy programs requiring physical attendance at weekly meetings. "Thus, the Internet appears to be a viable method for delivery of structured behavioral weight loss programs deserving of future research," they write.[15]

Of course, this was a highly structured program, in a hospital Web site, designed by weight loss specialists. Whether this success rate would carry over to the diet plans that seem to pop up all over the

Web is another question. Our impression is that the quality of these programs is uneven (see sidebar, "Weight Control and the Internet").

Behavioral Research

Of course, we would not need a whole new shelf full of designer drugs or food substitutes if only more of us were capable of understanding, and emulating, the self-initiated changes that have been made by a number of formerly obese people. In chapter 3, we discussed the National Weight Control Registry, a database of people who have lost 60 pounds or more, and more important, have been able to keep it off for 5 years or more. One of the keepers of that registry, Dr. James Hill of the University of Colorado Health Sciences Center, says four common elements are integral to these slim-down champions' long-term success:

> ### Weight Control and the Internet
>
> As an experiment, we signed on for three of the most popular diet- or fitness-related commercial Web sites recently. We thought it would be revealing to see what kind of advice would be offered—not just to a person who is obese but to someone who really should not lose weight but instead gain weight. Larry entered a weight and height corresponding to a BMI of 15 (emaciated); he asked how he could lose 5 pounds. The two diet-focused sites surveyed suggested the following:
>
> **eDiets.com.** Larry was a perfect candidate for the eDiets program but should use a weight *maintenance* rather than weight *loss* diet.
>
> **DietSmart.com.** Larry should not lose even a pound.
>
> Neither program contradicted Larry's request enough to suggest that Larry should try to *gain* weight, nor did either suggest seeking

- Most of them follow a low-fat, high-carbohydrate diet.
- Most of them eat a daily breakfast.
- Most of them keep a close eye on themselves. They weigh themselves regularly and record their weight. They also keep a food journal. Some have maintained these habits for as long as 20 years after their initial weight loss.
- Most of them not only meet but exceed the recommended 30 minutes a day of physical activity. More than 90 percent get at least 1 hour of exercise a day. About three in four do it by walking.

It is safe to say that in the coming years, we will encounter more and more publicity about these successful habits. These are free changes, available to almost everyone with virtually no side effects, and they are proven to work.

---

professional help, despite clear signs of a possible eating disorder. Of the two, the DietSmart program seemed more individualized. eDiets had a number of typographic errors in its material, and neither seemed to have a medical adviser on its Web site. The range of on-line support groups seemed best at eDiets.

A third site, biogenesis.net, is principally a fitness rather than a weight-control site and was the most blatantly commercial of the three, with pop-up ads and a pill for sale with eight "magical" ingredients (but ephedrine, discussed in chapter 6, was not one of them).

The bottom line, in our opinion, is that in-person commercial programs such as Weight Watchers or TOPS (Take Off Pounds Sensibly) are a better value and likely to be more satisfying than an entirely online experience. For those who seek help and want anonymity, DietSmart.com seems the best of the bunch and may be worth a try.

"To keep lost weight off, people must change their approach to exercise and develop new habits," Dr. Hill said at a media briefing on obesity and weight loss sponsored by the American Medical Association. "People on weight maintenance need to exercise for about an hour a day, as opposed to the surgeon general's recommendation of 30 minutes a day at least 3 days a week. In addition to their daily routines of planned exercise such as walking, biking and lifting weights, I recommend people choose to be more active whenever they have the opportunity. For instance, walking up the stairs burns more calories than taking the elevator."[16]

In a series of publications written with his codirector, Dr. Rena Wing, and other researchers, Dr. Hill has provided equally fascinating insights into the attributes of long-term weight loss—and what distinguishes success from failure.

Despite the fact that many believe "almost no one" can take off large amounts of weight and keep it off, Drs. Hill and Wing say that more than 20 percent of obese people can lose weight successfully.

> Researchers found that less attention and less effort were required the longer the weight loss lasted.

The key, they say, is understanding what constitutes success in weight loss: shedding at least 10 percent of your initial body weight and keeping it off for 1 year or more.[17] In a study that will be encouraging to many in the early stages of weight loss, involving more than 900 people who had lost 30 pounds or more and kept the weight off for at least 2 years, the researchers found that less attention and less effort were required the longer the weight loss lasted.[18] This may offer some insight into why the risk of relapse to obesity seems to decrease the longer weight loss is maintained.

Looked at the other way, another study of people who had achieved substantial weight loss discovered important differences between those who were able to maintain their loss and those who relapsed. Those who regained weight had lost greater quantities of weight initially and also recorded greater levels of depression and binge eating when they were first logged into the registry. They maintained lower activity levels and consumed a greater percentage of fat in their diets than those who were able to maintain their weight loss.[19] In many respects, successful long-term weight-losers are fighting the same obstacles and background as those who try and fail. Two-thirds of those in the registry were overweight as children; more than half (60 percent) say they have a history of obesity in their families; and about half accomplished their weight reduction through their own solo effort—without the benefit of any structured program.[20] It really can be done, though the effort required is usually substantial. University of Minnesota researchers Nancy Sherwood and Robert Jeffery have suggested that more people might be convinced to adopt regular exercise programs if they understood that physical activity is good for us emotionally (it fights stress and helps to alleviate depression) and has been shown to help people stop smoking, as well as being an excellent way to maintain weight loss. "Exercise may also be a helpful strategy for individuals who are attempting to manage their use of other substances as well, such as alcohol or high-fat foods," they write. "Given the strong connection between physical activity and emotional well-being, more emphasis might be placed on promoting exercise as a stress management tool."[21]

> *More people might be convinced to adopt regular exercise programs if they understood that physical activity is good for us emotionally (it fights stress and helps to alleviate depression) and has been shown to help people stop smoking, as well as being an excellent way to maintain weight loss.*

The hardest part in combating the "epidemic of sedentariness" is reaching those individuals who are inactive and also have no positive experiences with exercise or any current intention to begin exercising, Sherwood and Jeffery acknowledge. Targeted communications may be necessary for such individuals, including, perhaps, direct mail campaigns, they suggest. As for the importance of involving others, research shows that social support—including spouses, friends, and exercise partners—is critical to exercise programs for many people. That point is particularly true of women, who often say that "social interaction" is of primary importance in their desire to exercise.

While the expressed desire to lose weight is widespread, another study suggests that many people have not gotten the message on what is needed to achieve it. Recent research from the Centers for Disease Control and Prevention found that only about one in five people who report trying to lose weight are *both* reducing their consumption of calories from all sources *and* getting the minimum prescribed level of 150 minutes of exercise per week. "Of particular concern was the finding that using physical activity as a method to lose weight was least common among the obese, the least educated, and the oldest," the researchers say. "This suggests a need for better communication by health-care professionals to facilitate the adoption of physical activity for weight control, especially among these groups."[22]

SOCIETAL CHANGES

As we noted in chapter 7, U.S. Surgeon General David Satcher has issued a "call to action" in the fight against overweight. Just by themselves, he warned, the nation's bulging waistlines could undo all the advances that have been made against cancer and heart disease in the war against smoking. That medical judgment may get fewer people's attention, however, than some of the specific action steps he has recommended. Many are aimed at children and teens, in the recognition that life patterns—and the predisposition for obesity—are set very early. Who knows—some of these activities may be coming soon to a neighborhood near you:

- All students, at all grades, should receive daily physical education. Surprisingly (at least for those of us over 40 who remember trying to hoist ourselves hand over hand up a rope and enduring other regular challenges in physical education), only one state—Illinois—currently requires PE in all grades, beginning in kindergarten and continuing through high school.
- Improve the healthfulness of the food selections available in school cafeterias. Make more low-fat and low-calorie foods available. Offer more fruits and vegetables. Enforce regulations from the U.S. Department of Agriculture that prohibit serving foods of "low nutritional value" during mealtimes in school cafeterias, including snack foods and sodas dispensed by many schools' vending machines.
- Cut down on the 2 hours a day or more that the average high schooler spends watching television.
- Encourage mothers to breast-feed their infants.
- Increase research into the roots of overweight and obesity.
- Try to understand better and change the racial and ethnic disparities that mean ethnic minorities and poor people are disproportionately represented in the ranks of the obese.[23]

> *Although it is true that individuals have to change and that we are all ultimately responsible for ourselves, it is also true that pervasive forces in our culture and economy reinforce our sedentary lifestyles.*

Although it is true that individuals have to change and that we are all ultimately responsible for ourselves, it is also true that pervasive forces in our culture and economy reinforce our sedentary lifestyles. In particular, our lives have become increasingly organized around the automobile and the prevalence and convenience of fast food.

"The most important piece that is missing is effective approaches by which communities can make it easier for people to get regular physical activity—to be physically active and to maintain a healthy body weight," says Dr. Michael Thun, vice president of epidemiology and surveillance research for the American Cancer Society. "Physical activity has become largely optional in the American lifestyle. We have engineered it out of the activities of daily living. What is needed is to engineer it back in. We need to motivate communities to think creatively about ways to do that—the kinds of things that work in Europe and cause the average person [there] to be more physically active.

"There's a lot more walking built into daily life [in Europe]," Dr. Thun continues. "The societies are not as car based, and they are not as dispersed. There are more places to walk and to ride bikes and to use up some of the calories that we take in. In this country, there are structural factors that make that more difficult.

"A second big thing," he adds, "is that portion size is heavily used to market both restaurant foods and fast foods. The all-you-can-eat concept is an effective marketing tool. It's a relatively inexpensive marketing tool because much of the cost is in the food preparation, not in the actual food volume. The consequence is that it encourages overeating. In fast-food restaurants, the largest beverage size may contain half of a person's daily caloric needs, and market research indicates that most people drink most of the drink before they leave the restaurant.

"Furthermore, the plate size in restaurants has increased dramatically over time. A chef pointed out to a colleague that the appetizer used to be served on a salad plate in the past, and now it's an 8- or 9-incher. The main course used to be served on an 8- or 9-inch plate in the past, and now it's a 15-incher."

As these examples indicate, the modern epidemic of obesity is tied into the warp and woof of American society. Traditional approaches, exhorting the individual reader or listener to get more exercise and eat less, have fallen on increasingly pudgy and largely deaf ears. Writing in the journal, *Public Health Reports*, researchers Marion Nestle and Michael Jacobson (from New York University and the Center for

Science in the Public Interest, respectively) list no fewer than 36 major policy statements by the federal government and major private health organizations between 1952 and 1999 intended to prevent obesity and promote healthy weight. "Typically, these guidelines focused on individuals and tended to state the obvious," they write. Despite the fact that obesity prevention "has been an explicit goal of national public health policy since 1980," they note, rates of overweight continued to climb nationally throughout the 1980s and 1990s. While reported caloric intake has risen in the past couple of decades, other trends have pointed downward: "The proportions of schools offering physical education, overweight people who report dieting and exercising to lose weight, and primary-care physicians who counsel patients about behavioral risk factors for obesity and other conditions have all declined."[24]

At the same time, Nestle and Jacobson note that the fast-food industry promotes its wares with budgets that dwarf the public health agencies' marketing campaigns: McDonald's alone spent more than $1 billion for promotion in 1998, compared with the mere $1 million per year spent by the National Cancer Institute to promote the 5-A-Day fruit and vegetable campaign or the $1.5 million budgeted by the National Heart, Lung, and Blood Institute for its National Cholesterol Education Campaign. The ubiquity of 170,000 fast-food restaurants and 3 million soda vending machines, along with steadily increasing portion sizes, "help explain why it requires more and more willpower for Americans to maintain an appropriate intake of energy," these researchers say.[25]

> *McDonald's alone spent more than $1 billion for promotion in 1998, compared with the mere $1 million per year spent by the National Cancer Institute to promote the 5-A-Day fruit and vegetable campaign or the $1.5 million budgeted by the National Heart, Lung, and Blood Institute for its National Cholesterol Education Campaign.*

Here are some of Nestle and Jacobson's suggested policy responses, which they consider amply warranted in view of the huge price tag of obesity-related diseases and deaths:

- Place small taxes on sodas and other high-fat, high-calorie, high-sugar foods, and spend the revenue generated that way on health education campaigns.
- Restrict commercials for sodas, snacks, and fast food on TV shows commonly watched by children under age 10.
- Require (and provide the funding for) daily physical education classes in both primary and secondary schools.
- Ban the sale of sodas, candy bars, and other high-calorie snack food in schools.
- On the municipal level, encourage walking and mass transit use; promote pedestrian malls and auto-free zones; and build more bicycle paths, swimming pools, and sidewalks to encourage walking. The authors suggest that small taxes on new televisions, cars, or gasoline could help to pay for these public improvements.[26]

One of these researchers' many recommendations—that the surgeon general issue a report on obesity prevention—came to pass only a year after they had published their article. The December 2001 report from Dr. David Satcher, while avoiding calls for increased taxation or restrictions on TV fast-food commercials aimed at children, does stress that many of the steps needed to address the obesity epidemic are a "community responsibility," not just personal matters.[27] Dr. Satcher supported research into the marketing practices of the fast-food industry; prohibition of vending machines that compete with school cafeterias in elementary schools, and restricted access to them in secondary schools; and evaluation of the contracts that many schools have with snack and soda companies to allow the placement of vending machines on school property.

Beyond that, Dr. Satcher called for a number of changes in the way obesity is viewed in the health-care community, beginning with the biggest, fuzziest, and most elusive goal of all—the goal to which most of this book has been devoted: "develop effective preventive and therapeutic programs for obesity." But some of the other proposed changes were more specific:

- Review the policies of both public (governmental) and private health insurers with respect to paying for obesity prevention as well as treatment.
- Begin discussing the idea of declaring obesity a disease with a reimbursement code for insurers.
- Encourage employers to establish fitness centers at the work site or to give their employees incentives to join fitness centers outside work.
- Give all employees "protected time" for lunch.
- "Promote and support breast-feeding" at work as a means of preventing obesity in children, as well as assisting mothers in returning to their prepregnancy weight (although the report does not explain how babies would fit into the average workplace).

Some of this 60-page report might seem impossibly idealistic. Maybe it is. But consider what was accomplished with regard to smoking tobacco. In 1965, 42 percent of all American adults smoked cigarettes. By 1999, after several decades of major antitobacco publicity led by a series of surgeons general as well as the Food and Drug Administration, that percentage had been whittled down to 24—a reduction of more than 40 percent.

> Although the message may be more complex, the bottom line is the same for obesity as it was for smoking. Overweight can make us sick.

Although the message may be more complex, the bottom line is the same for obesity as it was for smoking. Overweight can make us sick. It is possible that a clear focus on the dangers of bad diet and our sedentary lifestyle may produce the same results as the antismoking campaign. Suppose we could reverse the national gains of the past half-century and cut our rate of obesity by 40 percent or more.

The public health payoff would be vast—just as it was in smoking. Impossible? Implausible now, perhaps—but certainly possible.

The stakes are just as great.

Appendix: Resources

About Weight Loss
Web site: www.weightloss.about.com

Academy for Eating Disorders
Web site: www.aedweb.org

American Cancer Society
Web site: www.cancer.org

American Diabetes Association
Web site: www.diabetes.org

American Dietetic Association
National Center for Nutrition and Dietetics (NCND) Information Line
Phone: (800) 366-1655
Web site: www.eatright.org

American Heart Association
Phone: (800) 242-8721
Web site: www.americanheart.org

American Obesity Association
Phone: (800) 986-2373
Web site: www.obesity.org

American Society for Dermatologic Surgery
Phone: (847) 330-9830
Web site: www.asds-net.org

American Society of Plastic Surgeons
Phone: (888) 475-2784
Web site: www.plasticsurgery.org

Centers for Disease Control and Prevention
Web site: www.cdc.gov/nccdphp/dnpa/obesity/index.htm

Federal Trade Commission
The Facts About Weight Loss Products and Programs
Web site: http://vm.cfsan.fda.gov/~dms/wgtloss.html

Harvard Center for Cancer Prevention
Web site: www.yourcancerrisk.harvard.edu

InteliHealth
Diseases and Conditions/Weight Management
Web site: www.intelihealth.com

National Eating Disorders Association
Phone: (206) 382-3587
Web site: http://nationaleatingdisorders.org

National Heart, Lung, and Blood Institute
Obesity Education Initiative
Web site: www.nhlbi.nih.gov/about/oei/index.htm

National Task Force on Prevention and Treatment of Obesity
Web site: www.niddk.nih.gov/fund/divisions/DDN/obesitytaskforce.htm

National Institute of Diabetes and Digestive and Kidney Diseases (NIDDK)
Weight Control and Loss
Web site: www.niddk.nih.gov/health/nutrit/nutrit.htm

Pennington Biomedical Research Center
Louisiana State University
Web site: www.pbrc.edu

Quackwatch
Web site: www.quackwatch.com

The United States Department of Agriculture
Web site: www.usda.gov

FINDING A DOCTOR

American Board of Internal Medicine (Directory of Diplomates)
Web site: www.abim.org/dp/apps/physdir.htms

American College of Surgeons
Web site: www.facs.org/fellows_info/statements/st-34.html

American Medical Association Physician Select
Web site: www.ama-assn.org/aps/amahg.htm

American Society of Bariatric Physicians
Phone: (303) 779-4833
Web site: www.asbp.org/locate.htm

American Society for Bariatric Surgery
Phone: (352) 331-4900
Web site: www.asbs.org/html/member.html

UNIVERSITY WEIGHT-CONTROL PROGRAMS

Duke Diet and Fitness Program
804 West Trinity Avenue
Durham, NC 27701
Phone: (800) 235-3853
Web site: www.dukecenter.org

Johns Hopkins Weight Management Center
2360 West Joppa Road,
   Suites 205 and 300
Lutherville, MD 21093
Phone: (410) 847-3744
Web site: www.jhbmc.jhu.edu
   /weight

New York Obesity Research Center
St. Luke's–Roosevelt Hospital
1090 Amsterdam Avenue,
   14th Floor
New York, NY 10025
Phone: (212) 523-4196
Web site: http://cpmcnet.columbia
   .edu/dept/obesectr/NYORC

LifeLong Sustained Weight Loss Program
Stanford Center for Integrative
   Medicine
Stanford Hospital & Clinics
1101 Welch Road, Suite A6
Palo Alto, CA 94304
Phone: (650) 498-5566
Web site: www.stanfordhospital
   .com/clinicsmedServices
   /clinics/complementaryMedicine
   /scimLifeLongWeightLoss.html

Colorado Weigh 16-Week Weight Loss Program
University of Colorado Health
   Sciences Center
200 E. 9th Avenue
Campus Box C-225,
Denver, CO 80262
Phone: (303) 315-2602
Web site: www.uchsc.edu/colorado
   weigh/index.htm

Weight and Eating Disorders Program
University of Pennsylvania
3535 Market Street, Suite 3108
Philadelphia, PA 19104
Phone: (215) 898-7314
Web site: www.uphs.upenn.edu
   /~weight

Yale Center for Eating and Weight Disorders
P.O. Box 208205
New Haven, CT 06520
Phone: (203) 432-4610
Web site: www.yale.edu/ycewd

FURTHER READING

Better Homes and Gardens 3 Steps to Weight Loss by Lawrence J. Cheskin, M.D. (Meredith Books, 2001).

Fat: Fighting the Obesity Epidemic by Robert Pool (Oxford University Press, 2001).

Losing Weight for Good: Developing Your Personal Plan of Action by Lawrence J. Cheskin, M.D. (Johns Hopkins University Press, 2001).

The Volumetrics Weight-Control Plan: Feel Full on Fewer Calories by Barbara J. Rolls, Ph.D., and Robert A. Barnett (Quill, 2000).

PEDOMETER

To order the LEARN WalkMaster, an electronic pedometer that can measure your steps, the distance you have walked, and the calories you have burned, call 1-888-LEARN-41 or go to www.TheLifeStyleCompany.com on the Internet.

Notes

Chapter 1

1. "Obesity Epidemic Puts Millions at Risk from Related Diseases," World Health Organization, Press Release WHO/46, June 12, 1997, www.who.int/archives /inf-pr-1997/en/pr97-46.html, accessed June 19, 2001; and "Controlling the Global Obesity Epidemic," World Health Organization, www.who.int/nut/obs.htm, accessed June 19, 2001.
2. G.A. Bray, C. Bouchard, and W.P.T. James, "Definitions and Proposed Current Classification of Obesity," in *Handbook of Obesity*, ed. G.A. Bray, C. Bouchard, and W.P.T. James (New York: Dekker, 1998): 31–40.
3. T.A. Wadden and T. B. VanItallie, "Preface," in *Treatment of the Seriously Obese Patient*, ed. T.A. Wadden and T.B. VanItallie (New York: Guilford, 1992): *xii*.
4. "Pets Need to Count Calories Too, Says Texas A&M Vet," www.tamu.edu /univrel/aggiedaily/news/stories/00/072500-6.html, accessed September 18, 2001.
5. "Overweight Cats and Dogs: Causes, Risks, Treatment, Prevention," Pet Education.com, www.peteducation.com/nutrition/overweight.htm, accessed September 18, 2001.
6. "Obesity in Dogs" and "Obesity in Cats," www.purina.com/dogs/nutrition .asp?article=201, accessed September 18, 2001.
7. P.J. Brown and V.K. Bentley-Condit, "Culture, Evolution, and Obesity," in *Handbook of Obesity*: 143–155.
8. G.A. Bray, "Historical Framework for the Development of Ideas About Obesity," in *Handbook of Obesity*: 1–30.
9. R. Pool, *Fat: Fighting the Obesity Epidemic* (New York: Oxford University Press, 2001).
10. C. Bouchard, L. Perusse, T. Rice, and D.C. Rao, "The Genetics of Human Obesity," in *Handbook of Obesity*: 157–190.

11. K.M. Flegal, R.P. Troiano, E.R. Pamuk, R.J. Kuczmarski, and S.M. Campbell, "The Influence of Smoking Cessation on the Prevalence of Overweight in the United States," *New England Journal of Medicine* 333 (1995): 1165–1170.
12. National Institute of Diabetes and Digestive and Kidney Diseases, "Diet and Exercise Dramatically Delay Type 2 Diabetes: Diabetes Medication Metformin Also Effective," www.niddk.nih.gov/welcome/releases/8_8_01.htm, accessed August 9, 2001.
13. A.M. Wolf and G.A. Colditz, "Current Estimates of the Economic Cost of Obesity in the United States," *Obesity Research* 6 (1998): 97–106.
14. F.M. Cicuttini and F.M. Spector, "Obesity, Arthritis, and Gout," in *Handbook of Obesity*: 741–752.
15. American Cancer Society, "Cancer Facts & Figures 2001."
16. Z. Huang et al., "Dual Effects of Weight and Weight Gain on Breast Cancer Risk," *Journal of the American Medical Association* 278, no. 17 (1997): 1448–1449.
17. D.S. Coffey, "Similarities of Prostate and Breast Cancer: Evolution, Diet, and Estrogens," *Urology* 57, no. 4, supplement 1 (April 2001): 31–38.
18. D.S. Michaud et al., "Physical Activity, Obesity, Height, and the Risk of Pancreatic Cancer," *Journal of the American Medical Association* 286 (2001): 921–929.
19. National Heart, Lung, and Blood Institute, "Clinical Guidelines on the Identification, Evaluation, and Treatment of Overweight and Obesity in Adults—The Evidence Report," in *Obesity Research* 6, supplement 2 (September 1998).
20. The RAND Corporation, "Obesity Linked to Higher Rates of Chronic Illness and Worse Physical Quality of Life than Smoking, Drinking, or Poverty: Three of Five Adult Americans Are Overweight or Obese," June 7, 2001.
21. S.K. Fried and C.D. Russell, "Diverse Roles of Adipose Tissue in the Regulation of Systemic Metabolism and Energy Balance," in *Handbook of Obesity*: 397–413.
22. R. Weiss, "Human Fat May Provide Useful Cells," *Washington Post*, April 10, 2001: A-1.

Chapter 2

1. L.J. Cheskin, *Losing Weight for Good: Developing Your Personal Plan of Action* (Baltimore: Johns Hopkins University Press, 1997).

2. E.J. Drenick, G.S. Bale, F. Seltzer, and D.G. Johnson, "Excessive Mortality and Causes of Death in Morbidly Obese Men," *Journal of the American Medical Association* 243, no. 5 (1980): 443–445.
3. D. Grady, "The State of Weight: Many Are Too Fat for the Calipers," *New York Times*, www.nytimes.com/2001/01/09/health/09FAT.html, accessed January 9, 2001.
4. Centers for Disease Control and Prevention, "Obesity Continues Climb in 1999 Among American Adults," www.cdc.gov/nccdphp/dnpa/pr-obesity.htm. Accessed June 27, 2001.
5. G.A. Bray, "Classification and Evaluation of the Overweight Patient," in *Handbook of Obesity*, ed. G.A. Bray, C. Bouchard, and W.P.T. James (New York: Dekker, 1998): 831–854.
6. National Institute on Drug Abuse, "Therapy to Help Women Reduce Their Concerns About Gaining Weight Found to Be Effective in Helping Them to Stop Smoking," www.nida.nih.gov/MedAdv/01/NR8-1.html, accessed October 15, 2001.
7. D.A. Galuska et al., "Are Health Care Professionals Advising Obese Patients to Lose Weight?" *Journal of the American Medical Association* 282 (1999): 1576–1578.

Chapter 3

1. J.F. Munroe and I. Stolarek, "Very Low Calorie Diets: Future Perspectives," *International Journal of Obesity* 13 (1989): 11–15.
2. Committee on Medical Aspects of Food Policy, *Report of the Working Group on Very Low Calorie Diets: The Use of Very Low Calorie Diets in Obesity* (London: Her Majesty's Stationery Office, 1987).
3. J.W. Anderson, E.C. Konz, R.C. Frederich, and C.L. Wood, "Long-Term Weight-Loss Maintenance: A Meta-analysis of US Studies," *American Journal of Clinical Nutrition* 74, no. 5 (2001): 579–584.
4. National Institutes of Health/National Heart, Lung, and Blood Institute, "Clinical Guidelines on the Identification, Evaluation and Treatment of Overweight and Obesity in Adults," *Obesity Research* 6 (1998): 51S–209S.
5. American Dietetic Association, "Are You a Portion Size Dropout? ADA Offers Visual Aids to Cure Portion Distortion," press release, 1999; and "Portion Sizes You'll Understand," www.eatright.org, accessed October 20, 2001.
6. G.P. Ravelli, Z.A. Stein, and M.W. Susser, "Obesity in Young Men after Famine Exposure in Utero and Early Infancy," *New England Journal of Medicine* 295, no. 7 (1976): 349–353.

7. M. Schorr, "High-Fat Diets Trigger Changes in Brain Chemistry," Reuters Health, September 13, 2001, www.reutershealth.com, accessed September 18, 2001.
8. National Weight Control Registry, www.uchsc.edu/nutrition/uwcr.htm, accessed October 20, 2001.
9. A. Fletcher and V.E. Brody, *Thin for Life: 10 Keys to Success From People Who Have Lost Weight and Kept It Off* (Boston: Houghton Mifflin, 1995).
10. *Dietary Guidelines for Americans, 2000*, 5th ed., www.usda.gov/cnpp/Pubs/DG2000/Index.htm.
11. S. Kayman, W. Bruvoid, and J.S. Stern, "Maintenance and Relapse After Weight Loss in Women: Behavioral Aspects," *American Journal of Clinical Nutrition* 52 (1990): 800–807.
12. E.T. Mannix, J.M. Dempsey, R.J. Engel, B. Schneider, and M.F. Busk, "The Role of Physical Activity, Exercise, and Nutrition in the Treatment of Obesity," in D.J. Goldstein, ed., *The Management of Eating Disorders and Obesity* (Humana Press, Totowa, NJ, 1999): 155.
13. Ibid., p. 166.
14. K.D. Brownell, *The LEARN Program for Weight Management 2000* (American Health Publishing Company, Dallas, Texas, 2000): 20.
15. G. Alan Marlatt and Judith Gordo, *Relapse Prevention* (Guilford Press, New York, 1985).

Chapter 4

1. S.C. Woods, "Food Intake and the Regulation of Body Weight," *Annual Review of Psychology*, 2000, www.findarticles.com/cf_0/m0961/2000_Annual/61855628/print.jhtml, accessed June 22, 2001.
2. K.M. Gadde, C.B. Parker, L.G. Maner, H.R. Wagner, E.J. Logue, M.K. Drezner, and K.R.R. Krishnan, "Bupropion for Weight Loss: An Investigation of Efficacy and Tolerability in Overweight and Obese Women," *Obesity Research* 9 (2001): 544–551.
3. L.M. Dickerson and P.J. Carek, "Drug Therapy for Obesity," *American Family Physician*, April 1, 2000, www.aafp.org/afp/20000401/2131.html, accessed January 18, 2001.
4. National Institute of Diabetes and Digestive and Kidney Diseases, "Prescription Medications for the Treatment of Obesity," www.niddk.nih.gov/health/nutrit/pubs/presmeds.htm, accessed January 18, 2001.

5. L.K. Khan, M.K. Serdula, B.A. Bowman, and D.F. Williamson, "Use of Prescription Weight Loss Pills Among U.S. Adults in 1996–1998," *Annals of Internal Medicine* 134, no. 4 (2001): 282–286.

6. National Institute of Diabetes and Digestive and Kidney Diseases, "Prescription Medications for the Treatment of Obesity," www.niddk.nih.gov/health/nutrit/pubs/presmeds.htm, accessed January 18, 2001.

7. Ibid.

8. M. Agrawal, M. Worzniak, and L. Diamond, "Managing Obesity Like Any Other Chronic Condition: Long-Term Therapy May Reduce Comorbidity as Well," *Postgraduate Medicine* 108 (2000), www.postgradmed.com/issues/2000/07_00/agrawal.htm, accessed August 1, 2001.

9. G. Glazer, "Long-Term Pharmacotherapy of Obesity 2000: A Review of Efficacy and Safety," *Archives of Internal Medicine* 161 (2001): 1814–1824.

10. W.P. James, A. Astrup, N. Finer, J. Hilsted, P. Kopelman, S. Rossner, W.H. Saris, and L.F. Van Gaal, "Effect of Sibutramine on Weight Maintenance After Weight Loss: A Randomized Trial: STORM Study Group, Sibutramine Trial of Obesity Reduction and Maintenance," *The Lancet* 356, no. 9248 (December 23–30, 2000): 2119–2125.

11. J.P. Després, "Drug Treatment for Obesity: We Need More Studies in Men at Higher Risk of Coronary Events," *British Medical Journal* 322 (2001): 1379–1380.

12. Glazer, "Long-Term Pharmacotherapy of Obesity 2000."

13. Ibid.

14. H.M. Connolly, J.L. Crary, M.D. McGoon, D.D. Hensrud, B.S. Edwards, W.D. Edwards, and H.V. Schaff, "Valvular Heart Disease Associated with Fenfluramine-Phentermine," *New England Journal of Medicine* 337, no. 9 (1997): 581–588.

15. M.A. Khan, C.A. Herzog, J.V. St. Peter, G.G. Hartley, R. Madlon-Kay, C.D. Dick, R.W. Asinger, and J.T. Vessey, "The Prevalence of Cardiac Valvular Insufficiency Assessed by Transthoracic Echocardiography in Obese Patients Treated with Appetite-Suppressant Drugs," *New England Journal of Medicine* 339, no. 11 (1998): 765–766; and D.A. Anderson and T.A. Wadden, "Treating the Obese Patient: Suggestions for Primary Care Practice," *Archives of Family Medicine* 8 (1999): 156–167.

16. Glazer, 2001.

17. T.A. Wadden, R.I., Berkowitz, D.B. Sarwer, R. Prus-Wisniewski, and C. Steinberg, "Benefits of Lifestyle Modification in the Pharmacologic Treatment of Obesity," *Archives of Internal Medicine* 161 (2001): 218–227.

Chapter 5

1. R.J. Albrecht and W.J. Pories, "Surgical Intervention for the Severely Obese," *Ballière's Clinical Endocrinology and Metabolism* 13, no. 1 (1999): 149.
2. J.S. Torgerson and L. Sjostrom, "The Swedish Obese Subjects (SOS) Study—Rationale and Results," *International Journal of Obesity Related Metabolic Disorders* (May 2001): S2–S4.
3. E. Leffler, S. Gustavsson, and B.M. Karlson, "Time Trends in Obesity Surgery 1987 Through 1996 in Sweden—A Population-Based Study," *Obesity Surgery* 10, no. 6 (December 2000): 543–548.
4. American College of Surgeons, "Recommendations for Facilities Performing Bariatric Surgery," *Bulletin of the American College of Surgeons* 85, no. 9 (September 2000): 9, www.facs.org/fellows_info/statements/st-34.html.
5. F. Charatan, "Obesity Surgery Grows in Popularity in the U.S.," *British Medical Journal* 321 (October 21, 2000): 980.
6. NIH Consensus Statement, "Gastrointestinal Surgery for Severe Obesity," 9, no. 1 (March 25–27, 1991): 1–20, http://text.nlm.nih.gov/nih/cdc/www/84txt.html, accessed September 27, 2001.
7. American Society for Bariatric Surgery, "Rationale for the Surgical Treatment of Morbid Obesity," www.asbs.org/html/ration.html, accessed September 5, 2001.
8. American Society for Bariatric Surgery, "The Story of Surgery for Obesity," www.asbs.org/html/story/ch_1.htm, accessed September 5, 2001.
9. Ibid.
10. Ibid.
11. Johns Hopkins Bayview Medical Center, Health Education Information, "Gastric Bypass Surgery for Obesity Surgery," undated report, provided September 7, 2001, by Dr. Thomas Magnuson; and National Institute of Diabetes and Digestive and Kidney Diseases, *Gastric Surgery for Severe Obesity*, NIH Publication No. 96-4006 (Washington, D.C.: Government Printing Office, April 1996).
12. American Society for Bariatric Surgery, "The Story of Surgery for Obesity."
13. National Institutes of Health; National Heart, Lung and Blood Institute; NHLBI Obesity Education Initiative; and North American Association for the Study of Obesity, *The Practical Guide: Identification,*

Evaluation, and Treatment of Overweight and Obesity in Patients, NIH Publication Number 00-4084 (Washington, D.C.: Government Printing Office, October 2000): 38.

14. National Institute of Diabetes and Digestive and Kidney Diseases, *Gastric Surgery for Severe Obesity*.
15. American Society for Bariatric Surgery, "The Story of Surgery for Obesity."
16. J.G. Kral, "Surgical Treatment of Obesity," in *Handbook of Obesity*, ed. G.A. Dray, C. Bouchard, and W.P.T. James (New York: Dekker, 1998): 988.
17. R.J. Albrecht and W.J. Pories, "Surgical Intervention for the Severely Obese," *Ballière's Clinical Endocrinology and Metabolism* 13, no. 1 (1999): 165.
18. Ibid., 155.
19. Dr. Charles Callery, personal interview; and www.thinnertimes.com, September 20, 2001.
20. Ibid.
21. Kral, "Surgical Treatment of Obesity," in *Handbook of Obesity*, 987–988.
22. Ibid., 988.
23. Albrecht and Pories, "Surgical Intervention for the Severely Obese," 159.
24. Ibid., 157.
25. D.G. Schultz, deputy director for clinical and review policy, Food and Drug Administration, approval letter to Ellen Duke, president and CEO, BioEnterics Corporation, June 5, 2001.
26. B.A. Schwetz, "New Weight-Reduction System," *Journal of the American Medical Association* 286, no. 5 (August 1, 2001); and FDA Talk Paper, "FDA Approves Implanted Stomach Band to Treat Severe Obesity," www.fda.gov/bbs/topics/ANSWERS/2001/ANS01087.html, accessed June 5, 2001.
27. American Society of Plastic Surgeons, "2000 National Plastic Surgery Statistics: Cosmetic and Reconstructive Plastic Surgery," www.plasticsurgery.org, accessed September 10, 2001.
28. American Society for Dermatologic Surgery, "Liposuction Surgery," www.asds-net.org/lipo_surgery.html, accessed September 10, 2001.
29. American Society for Plastic Surgery, "Liposuction," www.plasticsurgery.org/surgery/lipo.htm, accessed September 10, 2001.

Chapter 6

1. Yahoo!, dir.yahoo.com/Business_and_Economy/Shopping_and_Services/Health/Weight_Loss/Products, accessed January 18, 2001.

2. G. Winter, "Fraudulent Marketers Capitalize on Demand for Sweat-Free Diets," *New York Times*, October 29, 2000, www.nytimes.com/2000/10/29/science/29DIET.html, accessed January 18, 2001.
3. A. Weil, "Chitosan for Weight Loss?" November 17, 1999, www.drweil.com/archiveqa/0,2283,1671,00.html, accessed October 1, 2001.
4. A. Weil, "What's Up with *The Zone*?" June 11, 1996, www.drweil.com/archiveqa /0,2283,18,00.html, accessed October 1, 2001.
5. Federal Trade Commission, "Advertising Cases Involving Weight Loss Products and Services 1927–April 1997," www.ftc.gov/opa/1997/9703/dietcase.htm, accessed November 7, 2001.
6. Federal Trade Commission, "Weight Watchers and Jenny Craig to Face Litigation over FTC Deceptive Advertising Charges: Nutri/System, Physicians Weight Loss Centers and Diet Center to Settle Similar Charges," www.ftc.gov/opa/predawn/F93/commdiet.htm, accessed November 7, 2001.
7. Adapted from Federal Trade Commission, "Skinny on Dieting," www.ftc.gov/bcp/conline/pubs/health/diets.htm, accessed November 7, 2001.
8. E. Cooper, "Ashtanga Yoga" and "Striptease Aerobics," *Us Weekly* (October 1, 2001): 55.
9. National Center for Complementary and Alternative Medicine, "Major Domains of Complementary and Alternative Medicine," http://nccam.nih.gov/nccam/fcp/classify/index.html, accessed October 26, 2001.
10. Adapted from National Center for Complementary and Alternative Medicine, "Approaching Complementary and Alternative Therapies," http://nccam.nih.gov/nccam/fcp/faq/considercam.html, accessed October 26, 2001.
11. American Society of Clinical Hypnosis, "How to Find a Hypnotherapist," www.asch.net/find.htm, accessed September 10, 2001.
12. Division of Psychological Hypnosis, American Psychological Association, cited in "Hypnosis for the Seriously Curious," www.hypnosis-research.org /hypnosis/serious.html, accessed October 26, 2001.
13. "Lose Weight with Hypnosis," advertisement, *The Frederick* (Maryland) *Post*, October 17, 2001: A-7.
14. J. Stradling, D. Roberts, A. Wilson, and F. Lovelock, "Controlled Trial of Hypnotherapy for Weight Loss in Patients with Obstructive Sleep Apnea," *International Journal of Obesity and Related Metabolic Disorders* 22, no. 3 (1998): 278–281.

15. C.H. Haber, R. Nitkin, and I.R. Shenker, "Adverse Reactions to Hypnotherapy in Obese Adolescents: A Developmental Viewpoint," *Psychiatric Quarterly* 51, no. 1 (1979): 55–63.

16. D.B. Allison and M.S. Faith, "Hypnosis as an Adjunct to Cognitive-Behavioral Psychotherapy for Obesity: A Meta-analytic Reappraisal," *Journal of Consulting and Clinical Psychology* 64(3) (1996): 513–516.

17. Q. Sun and Y. Xu, "Simple Obesity and Obesity Hyperlipemia Treated with Otoacupoint Pellet Pressure and Body Acupuncture," *Journal of Traditional Chinese Medicine* 13, no. 1 (1993): 22–26.

18. Z. Liu, F. Sun, J. Li, Y. Han, Q. Wei, and C. Liu, "Application of Acupuncture and Moxibustion for Keeping Shape," *Journal of Traditional Chinese Medicine* 18, no. 4 (1998): 265–271.

19. Acupuncture Information and Resources, National Center for Complementary and Alternative Medicine, http://nccam.nih.gov/nccam/fcp/factsheets/acupuncture/acupuncture.htm, accessed October 26, 2001.

20. R.C. Niemtzow, J.R. Little, M.A. Matanga, B. Ferrer, J. Corn, and W. Kitto, "A High-Protein Regimen and Auriculomedicine for the Treatment of Obesity: A Second Clinical Observation," *Medical Acupuncture* 10, no. 2 (1998/1999), www.medicalacupuncture.org/aama_marf/journal/vol10_2/obesity.html, accessed October 26, 2001.

21. S.H.P. International Pty Ltd, "Proven Method for Weight Loss," www.shpinternational.com.au/acuslim.html, accessed November 5, 2001.

22. D. Richards and J. Marley, "Stimulation of Auricular Acupuncture Points in Weight Loss," *Australian Family Physician* 27, supplement 2 (1998): S73–S77.

23. R. Mazzoni, E. Mannucci, S.M. Rizzello, V. Ricca, and C.M. Rotella, "Failure of Acupuncture in the Treatment of Obesity: A Pilot Study," *Eating and Weight Disorders* 4, no. 4 (1999): 198–202.

24. E. Ernst, "Acupuncture/Acupressure for Weight Reduction? A Systematic Review," *Wiener Klinische Wochenschrift* 109, no. 2 (1997): 60–62.

25. M.A. Fobi, "Operations That Are Questionable for Control of Obesity," *Obesity Surgery* 3, no. 2 (1993): 197–200.

26. American Academy of Medical Acupuncture, "Interview with Dr. Jeff Baird," August 17, 2000, www.medicalacupuncture.org/acu_info/interviews/baird.html, accessed October 26, 2001.

27. Federal Trade Commission, Bureau of Protection, The American Society for Clinical Nutrition, The National Institute of Diabetes and Digestive and Kidney Diseases, The Centers for Disease Control and Prevention,

"Commercial Weight Loss Products and Programs: What Consumers Stand to Gain and Lose: A Public Conference on the Information Consumers Need to Evaluate Weight Loss Products and Programs," www.ftc.gov/os/1998/9803/weightlo.rpt.htm, accessed September 18, 2001.

28. Nanci Hellmich, "Bloom is off herbal-product sales," *USA Today*, August 13, 2001, www.usatoday.com/news/health/2001-05-09-herb-sale.htm, accessed September 18, 2001.

29. "Dexatrim Supplements, Natural Weight Loss for a Healthy Lifestyle," Product Information, Dexatrim Natural Green Tea Formula, www.dexatrim.com/product_science.asp, accessed October 1, 2001.

30. Food and Drug Administration, Federal Register 65 FR 17474-17477, April 3, 2000, "Dietary Supplements Containing Ephedrine Alkaloids; Withdrawal in Part," http://vm.cfsan.fda.gov/~lrd/fr00043a.html, accessed November 12, 2001.

31. R. Rubin, "Consumer Group: FDA Must Ban Ephedra," *USA Today*, September 5, 2001, www.usatoday.com/news/healthscience/health/2001-09-06-ephedra-usat.htm, accessed October 23, 2001.

32. Health Canada, "Advisory Not to Use Products Containing Ephedra or Ephedrine," June 14, 2001, www.hc-sc.gc.ca/english/archives/warnings/2001/2001_67e.htm, accessed October 1, 2001.

33. S. Squires, "The Risks of Fat Busters," *Washington Post*, March 28, 2000, HE14, www.washingtonpost.com/ac2/wp-dyn/A25452-2000Mar27?language=printer, accessed June 14, 2001.

34. L.J. Cheskin, "Ask the Expert," July 15, 2000, www.intelihealth.com, accessed October 13, 2001.

35. R. Guerciolini, L. Radu-Radulescu, M. Boldrin, J. Dallas, and R. Moore, "Comparative Evaluation of Fecal Fat Excretion Induced by Orlistat and Chitosan," *Obesity Research* 9 (2001): 364–367.

36. M.H. Pittler, N.C. Abbot, E.F. Harkness, and E. Ernst, "Randomized, Double-blind Trial of Chitosan for Body Weight Reduction," *European Journal of Clinical Nutrition* 53, no. 5 (1999): 379–381.

37. Federal Trade Commission, "Marketers of 'The Enforma System' Settle FTC Charges of Deceptive Advertising for Their Weight Loss Products," April 26, 2000, www.quackwatch.com/02ConsumerProtection/FTCActions/enforma.html, accessed October 1, 2001.

38. P. Kurtzweil, "Dieter's Brews Make Tea Time a Dangerous Affair," *FDA Consumer* (July–August 1997), www.fda.gov/fdac/features/1997/597_tea.html, accessed October 1, 2001.

39. U.S. Food and Drug Administration, Center for Food Safety and Applied Nutrition, "FDA Warns Consumers to Discontinue Use of Botanical Products That Contain Aristolochic Acid," April 11, 2001, www.cfsan.fda.gov/~dms/addsbot.html, accessed August 31, 2001.
40. H.M. Blanck, L.K. Khan, and M.K. Serdula, "Use of Nonprescription Weight Loss Products, Results from a Multistate Survey," *Journal of the American Medical Association* 286, no. 8 (2001): 930–935.

Chapter 7

1. R. Atkinson, "Etiologies of Obesity," in *The Management of Eating Disorders and Obesity*, ed. D.J. Goldstein (Totowa, NJ: Humana, 1999): 90.
2. D.J. Goldstein, "Foreword," in *The Management of Eating Disorders and Obesity:* ix.
3. Atkinson, "Etiologies of Obesity," in *The Management of Eating Disorders and Obesity:* 91.
4. D.A. Williamson and P.M. O'Neil, "Behavioral and Psychological Correlates of Obesity," in *Handbook of Obesity*, ed. G.A. Bray, C. Bouchard, and W.P.T. James (New York: Dekker, 1998): 130.
5. S.J. Romano, "Anorexia Nervosa," in *The Management of Eating Disorders and Obesity:* 51.
6. Ibid., 53.
7. Ibid., 51–52; also see S. Z. Yanovski, "Obesity and Eating Disorders," in *Handbook of Obesity:* 118.
8. C.L. Rock, "Prevention of Anorexia Nervosa and Bulimia Nervosa: A Nutritional Perspective," in *The Management of Eating Disorders and Obesity:* 35.
9. S.J. Romano, "Bulimia Nervosa," in *The Management of Eating Disorders and Obesity:* 9.
10. Ibid., 7.
11. M.D. Marcus, "Obese Patients with Binge-Eating Disorder," in *The Management of Eating Disorders and Obesity:* 125.
12. G.F. Adami, P. Gandolfo, B. Bauer, and N. Scopinaro, "Binge Eating in Massively Obese Patients Undergoing Bariatric Surgery," *International Journal of Eating Disorders* 17, no. 1 (January 1995): 45–50.
13. Marcus, "Obese Patients with Binge-Eating Disorder": 126.
14. S.Z. Yanovski, "Obesity and Eating Disorders," in *Handbook of Obesity:* 118.
15. National Task Force on the Prevention and Treatment of Obesity, "Dieting and the Development of Eating Disorders in Overweight and Obese Adults," *Archives of Internal Medicine* 160 (2000): 2581–2589.

16. M.E. Gluck, A. Geliebter, and T. Satov, "Night Eating Syndrome Is Associated with Depression, Low Self-Esteem, Reduced Daytime Hunger, and Less Weight Loss in Obese Outpatients," *Obesity Research* 9 (2001): 264–267.

17. L.K.G. Hsu, "Treatment of Anorexia Nervosa," in *The Management of Eating Disorders and Obesity:* 59, 67.

18. C.M. Grilo and R.M. Masheb, "Childhood Psychological, Physical, and Sexual Maltreatment in Outpatients with Binge Eating Disorder: Frequency and Associations with Gender, Obesity, and Eating-Related Psychopathology," *Obesity Research* 9, no. 5 (2001): 320–325.

19. American Obesity Association, "IRS Figures Weight Loss Programs into Tax Deductible Medical Expenses," December 18, 2000, www.obesity.org/irspress.htm, accessed October 16, 2001.

20. American Obesity Association, "A Taxpayer's Guide on IRS Policy to Deduct Weight Control Treatment," www.obesity.org/taxguide.htm, accessed October 16, 2001.

21. Internal Revenue Service, "Publication 502, Medical and Dental Expenses: What Medical Expenses Are Deductible?" www.irs.gov/prod/forms_pubs/pubs/p50205.htm, accessed October 16, 2000; and American Obesity Association, "IRS Figures."

22. D. Satcher, *The Surgeon General's Call to Action to Prevent and Decrease Overweight and Obesity: Overweight in Children and Adolescents*, www.surgeongeneral.gov/topics/obesity/calltoaction/fact_adolescents.htm, accessed December 16, 2001.

23. R. Strauss and H. Pollack, "Epidemic Increase in Childhood Overweight, 1986–1998," *Journal of the American Medical Association* 286 (2001): 2845–2848.

24. Satcher, *The Surgeon General's Call to Action*.

25. Centers for Disease Control and Prevention, National Center for Chronic Disease Prevention and Health Promotion, "Body Mass Index-for-Age," www.cdc.gov/nccdphp/dnpa/bmi/bmi-for-age.htm, accessed October 24, 2001.

26. American Obesity Association, 2000, "Healthy Weight 2010: Objectives for Achieving and Maintaining a Healthy Population": 15; and American Obesity Association, 2000, "Executive Summary: American Obesity Association Survey of Parental Attitudes on Their Children's Weight": 1.

27. D.S. Ludwig, K.E. Peterson, and S.L. Gortmaker, "Relation Between Consumption of Sugar-Sweetened Drinks and Childhood Obesity:

A Prospective, Observational Analysis," *The Lancet* 357, no. 9255 (2001): 505–508.
28. W.H. Dietz, "Prevalence of Obesity in Children," in *Handbook of Obesity*: 98–99.
29. American Medical Association, "Media Briefings: Overweight Children Risk Coronary Heart Disease and Diabetes as Obese Adults," July 12, 2001, www.ama-assn.org/ama/pub/article/4197-5160.html, accessed January 1, 2002.
30. American Obesity Association, "Obese Children Disliked More Today Than 40 Years Ago," press release, November 8, 2001.
31. Satcher, *The Surgeon General's Call to Action*.

Chapter 8
1. D.F. Phillips, "Leptin Passes Safety Tests, but Effectiveness Varies," *Journal of the American Medical Association* 280, no. 10 (1998): 869–870.
2. J.A. Yanovski and S.Z. Yanovski, "Recent Advances in Basic Obesity Research," *Journal of the American Medical Association* 282, no. 16 (1999): 1504.
3. S.B. Heymsfield et al., "Recombinant Leptin for Weight Loss in Obese and Lean Adults," *Journal of the American Medical Association* 282, no. 16 (1999): 1568–1575.
4. Phillips, "Leptin Passes Safety Tests": 870.
5. Yanovski and Yanovski, "Recent Advances in Basic Obesity Research": 1506.
6. Johns Hopkins Medical Institutions, "Compound That Switches Off Appetite in Mice Discovered by Hopkins Scientists," www.hopkinsmedicine.org/press/2000/JUNE/000629A.HTM, accessed January 4, 2002; also see Johns Hopkins Medical Institutions, "Experimental Appetite Suppressant Affects Numerous Brain Messengers In Mice," www.hopkinsmedicine.org/press/2002/JANUARY/020108A.htm.
7. Baylor College of Medicine, "Enzyme Could Provide Continual Fat Burning," http://public.bcm.tmc.edu/pa/fatburner.htm, accessed January 4, 2002.
8. Regeneron, "Axokine," http://graphics.regeneron.com/research/, accessed January 4, 2002.
9. D.F. Williamson, "Pharmacotherapy for Obesity," *Journal of the American Medical Association* 281, no. 3 (1999): 279.
10. BioEnterics Corporation, "The BIB System Alternative," www.bioenterics.com/intl/patient/bib/index.html, accessed September 7, 2001.

11. Transneuronix, www.transneuronix.com/about.html, accessed January 3, 2002.
12. V.V. Cigaina, A. Saggioro, V.V. Rigo, G. Pinato, and S. Ischai, "Long-Term Effects of Gastric Pacing to Reduce Feed Intake in Swine," *Obesity Surgery* 6, no. 3 (1996): 250–253.
13. R.L. Atkinson, "Etiologies of Obesity," in *The Management of Eating Disorders and Obesity*, ed. D.J. Goldstein (Totowa, NJ: Humana, 1999): 83–92.
14. N.V. Dhurandhar, B.A. Israel, J.M. Kolesar, G.F. Mayhew, M.E. Cook, and R.L. Atkinson, "Increased Adiposity in Animals Due to a Human Virus," *International Journal of Obesity and Related Metabolic Disorders* 24, no. 8 (2000): 989–996.
15. D.F. Tate, R.R. Wing, and R.A. Winett, "Using Internet Technology to Deliver a Behavioral Weight Loss Program," *Journal of the American Medical Association* 285, no. 9 (2001): 1172–1177.
16. American Medical Association, "Four Behaviors Identified That Can Spell Success in Maintaining Weight Loss," www.ama-assn.org/ama/pub/print/article/4197-5159.html, accessed January 1, 2002.
17. R.R. Wing and J.O. Hill, "Successful Weight Loss Maintenance," *Annual Reviews of Nutrition* 21 (2001): 323–341.
18. M.L. Klem, R.R. Wing, W. Lang, M.T. McGuire, and J.O. Hill, "Does Weight Loss Maintenance Become Easier over Time?" *Obesity Research* 8, no. 6 (2000): 438–444.
19. M.T. McGuire, R.R. Wing, M.L. Klem, W. Lang, and J.O. Hill, "What Predicts Weight Regain in a Group of Successful Weight Losers?" *Journal of Consulting and Clinical Psychology* 67, no. 3 (1999): 282.
20. University of Colorado Center for Human Nutrition, "National Weight Control Registry," www.uchsc.edu/nutrition/nwcr.htm, accessed August 9, 2001.
21. N.E. Sherwood and R.W. Jeffery, "The Behavioral Determinants of Exercise: Implications for Physical Activity Interventions," *Annual Reviews of Nutrition* 20 (2000): 21–44.
22. M.K. Serdula, A.H. Mokdad, D.F. Williamson, D.A. Galuska, J.M. Mendlein, and G.W. Heath, "Prevalence of Attempting Weight Loss and Strategies for Controlling Weight," *Journal of the American Medical Association* 282, no. 14 (1999): 1358.
23. U.S. Department of Health and Human Services, "Overweight and Obesity Threaten U.S. Health Gains: Communities Can Help Address the Problem, Surgeon General Says," press release, December 13, 2001.

24. M. Nestle and M.F. Jacobson, "Halting the Obesity Epidemic: A Public Health Policy Approach," *Public Health Reports* 115 (January/February 2000): 14, 16.
25. Ibid., 19
26. Ibid., 20–22.
27. U.S. Department of Health and Human Services, *The Surgeon General's Call to Action to Prevent and Decrease Overweight and Obesity 2001*, Public Health Service, Office of the Surgeon General, Rockville, Maryland (Washington, D.C.: Government Printing Office, 2001), www.surgeongeneral.gov/library.

Glossary

adipose tissue   Fatty tissue, composed of fat cells (adipocytes).

anorexia   Loss of appetite, as can be induced by most of the medications used in weight control, such as sibutramine and phentermine.

anorexia nervosa   An eating disorder characterized by distorted self-image and extreme thinness; can be life-threatening.

bariatrics   The field of medicine devoted to the treatment of obese persons.

bariatric surgery   Surgery for weight control, altering the passage of food through the stomach and small intestine.

bioimpedance   A way of measuring body composition by passing a tiny current through the body. Bioimpedance relies on the difference in electrical conductivity between fat, a poor electrical conductor, and lean tissue, a good conductor.

BMI   *See* Body Mass Index.

Body Mass Index (BMI)   The standard measure of obesity. Defined as weight in kilograms divided by the square of the height in meters. A BMI between 25 and 30 defines overweight; a BMI of 30 or more indicates obesity.

bulimia   An eating disorder characterized by consumption of great quantities of food in a short time, followed by vomiting or use of laxatives.

extreme obesity   Also called *morbid obesity*, a BMI of 40 or higher, which usually denotes a person is more than 100 pounds overweight.

fenfluramine   Anorexia-inducing drug that was withdrawn from the market in 1997 because of heart valve problems found in association with it. Fenfluramine was often used in combination with the drug phentermine, the so-called "fen-phen" combination. Phentermine was not found to be unsafe when used alone as directed.

gastric bypass A form of obesity surgery that involves restriction (forming a smaller stomach that fills up quickly) and bypassing the early portion of the small intestine (leading to poorer absorption of food calories).

gastric stapling or banding A form of obesity surgery that causes restriction by forming a smaller stomach pouch with staples or with a plastic band whose diameter can be adjusted.

hypothyroidism A disease in which the thyroid, a gland on the neck that helps to control the body's rate of metabolism, produces abnormally slow burning of calories. Hypothyroidism can be screened for with simple blood tests. It is the most common medically-treatable cause of obesity.

ideal body weight An older measure of relative weight; now sometimes referred to as *desirable body weight*.

laparoscopic surgery A newer means of performing operations that utilizes very small incisions through which instruments called laparoscopes are passed, allowing the surgeon to see, cut, and sew without requiring a large incision.

LCD *See* Low Calorie Diet.

leptin A recently-discovered hormone that plays a major role in controlling hunger and metabolism. Leptin is a small molecule that must be administered by injection rather than by mouth, and is undergoing testing as a treatment for some forms of obesity.

Low Calorie Diet (LCD) A diet containing at least 800 calories per day but fewer calories of energy than the individual is using. Thus, adherence to an LCD results in a moderate rate of weight loss.

morbid obesity *See* extreme obesity.

Obesity More than 25 percent of body weight comprised of adipose tissue for men and more than 30 percent for women; *or* a BMI of 30 or greater. *See also* Body Mass Index.

orlistat A drug for the treatment of obesity (brand name Xenical) that is not an appetite suppressant, but rather acts by blocking the digestion of about 30 percent of ingested fat calories.

overweight A lesser degree of excess adipose tissue than obesity; in the BMI range of 25 to 30. *See also* **Body Mass Index.**

phentermine   A drug for the treatment of obesity that is an appetite suppressant. It was the member of the "fen-phen" combination that was not found to be the problem and remains available for use.

sign   In medicine, any manifestation of a physical condition or disease that can be objectively measured or observed. Examples include a high blood pressure reading or a rash.

skinfold calipers   Instrument used to gently pinch the skin at specific locations, such as the abdomen, to yield a measure of fatness.

sleep apnea   A condition or syndrome characterized by poor sleep, snoring, and daytime sleepiness attributable to multiple, brief episodes of not breathing (apnea). Most patients with sleep apnea are extremelyobese. Also known as the Pickwickian syndrome.

symptom   In medicine, any manifestation of a physical condition or disease that is reported by a patient and is subjective. Examples include a complaint of headache or itching.

type 2 diabetes mellitus   A disease characterized by resistance to the effects of insulin, resulting in poor glucose utilization and a variety of symptoms, signs, and complications. Obesity is the leading cause of type 2 diabetes, and weight loss an effective treatment.

Very Low Calorie Diet (VLCD)   A diet containing fewer than 800 calories of energy per day. Adherence to a VLCD results in rapid weight loss and must be monitored medically.

VLCD   *See* Very Low Calorie Diet.

waist circumference   A measurement that when greater than 40 inches in men, or 36 inches in women, defines a form of obesity that confers particularly high health risks.

Index

A

Abdominal fat, 36, 45, 121
ACC2 blocker, 224–225
Acupuncture, 162, 171–175
Adipose cells, 28
Aerobic exercise, 103
African Americans, 10
Age, 39–40
Albrecht, Dr. R.J., 145, 150
Alcohol consumption, 15–16
Alternative and complementary
    treatments
  acupuncture, 162, 171–175
  aristolochic acid alert, 182–183
  choosing a practitioner, 168–169
  defined, 166–167
  FTC's list of no-no's, 164–165
  hypnotherapy, 167–171
  nonprescription drugs, 176–183
  summary on, 184–185
  warning regarding, 161–166
Aminorex, 110
Amphetamines, 110, 112, 114, 219
Anorexia nervosa, 188, 191–192, 196
Antidepressants, 16, 114
Appetite suppressants
  defined, 112
    phentermine, 115, 118, 119, 122, 123
    sibutramine (Meridia), 115, 118, 120, 122, 123, 124, 126
Aristolochic acid, 182–183

Atkinson, Dr. Richard L., 190, 229
Axokine, 225

B

Baird, Dr. Jeff, 175
Bariatric physicians, 55–56
Bariatric surgery
  benefits of, 144–145, 146
  candidates for, 133–136
  as choice of last resort, 129–130
  defined, 129
  food after, 150–151
  health insurance and, 151, 208, 209
  laparoscopically adjustable gastric
    band, 139, 151–154, 156–159
  liposuction following, 154–156, 209
  options for, 136–139
  overview, 130–132
  paying for, 151
  recommended standards, 140–141
  risks and side effects of, 139, 142–144
  rules to follow after, 148–149
  summary on, 159–160
  treatment after, 145–150
  Wayne Smith's story, 156–159
Behavioral issues, 105–108
Behavioral research, 232–236
Bentley-Condit, Vicki, 8
Berkowitz, Dr. Robert, 216
Biliopancreatic diversion (BPD), 139, 145

Binge eating disorder, 188–189, 194–195, 196
Bioelectrical impedance, 49
Bioenterics Intragastric Balloon (BIB), 226
Blood clots, 23–24
Body build, 39
Body fat distribution, 36, 37
Body fat tests, 48–50
Body Mass Index (BMI)
  children and, 211–214
  defined, 20, 42–45
  drug therapy and, 115
  obesity defined by, 26–27
  waist circumference and, 46–47, 48
Bray, George, 1, 9
Breast cancer (postmenopausal), 18, 24–25
Breast-feeding, 39, 118, 237, 241
Brown, Peter, 8
Brownell, Kelly, 104
Bulimia nervosa, 188, 193–194
Bupropion (Wellbutrin or Zyban), 114
Burkholder, Dr. William J., 6

C

C75 compound, 224
Caffeine
  ephedrine and, 112, 177, 179, 180
  as stimulant, 112, 113
Callery, Dr. Charles, 147, 148
Caloric compensation, 227
Calories
  awareness of, 89
  body's need for, 84
  counting, 83, 93
  exercise for burning, 87, 101–102
  in food-based plans, 90
  Low Calorie Diets (LCDs), 75–79
  Very Low Calorie Diets (VLCDs), 71–75, 110
Cancer, 18, 24–26
Carpenter, Karen, 191

Causes of obesity
  genetic diseases and disorders, 10, 12–14
  hypothalamus disorders, 10, 14–15
  lifestyle, 10, 11–12, 33
  medications, 10, 16
  smoking cessation, 10, 15, 51, 52–53, 112
Child abuse, 189, 197–198
Childhood obesity
  causes of, 212, 215
  consequences of, 216–217
  increase in, 209–211
  measurements for, 211–214
  prescriptions for, 217–218
Chitosan, 180–181
Cigarette smoking. *See* Smoking cessation
Coffey, Donald S., 25
Colon cancer, 18, 24, 25
Complementary and alternative treatments
  acupuncture, 162, 171–175
  aristolochic acid alert, 182–183
  choosing a practitioner, 168–169
  defined, 166–167
  FTC's list of no-no's, 164–165
  hypnotherapy, 167–171
  nonprescription drugs, 176–183
  summary on, 184–185
  warning regarding, 161–166
Cook, Dr. Curtiss, 216
Cushing's syndrome, 10, 13, 30

D

Després, Jean-Pierre, 121, 122
Dexatrim, 177–180
Dexfenfluramine (Redux), 118, 122, 123, 163
Diabetes, Type 2
  bariatric surgery and, 145, 146
  childhood obesity and, 210, 215, 216
  description of, 18, 19–20

Dexatrim and, 178
increase in, 19–20, 50
Joanna Givens' story, 30–33
Linda's story, 62–67, 188
liver disease and, 23
in Pima Indians, 10
as sign of obesity, 38, 97
Diagnosis
    body fat tests, 48–50
    Body Mass Index (BMI), 42–45, 211–214
    distribution of fat, 36, 37
    healthy weight ranges, 40, 41
    ideal body weight (IBW), 38–40, 73
    Linda's story, 62–67, 188
    medical evaluation, 51–57
    overweight versus obesity, 40, 42, 47
    risk factors, 50–51
    signs and symptoms, 37–38
    summary on, 68
    waist circumference, 45–47
    weight management clinics, 57–62
Dietary Supplement Health and Education Act of 1994 (DSHEA), 176–177
Diethylpropion (Tenuate), 113
Dietitians, 38, 60, 66
Diets
    defining success, 79–80
    fad dieting, 88–89
    food-based plans, 90–91
    how and when to weigh yourself, 81
    long-term success of, 91–94
    Low Calorie Diets (LCDs), 75–79
    new understanding of, 69–71
    plateauing, 80–84
    set point theory, 84–87
    successful methods, 87–90
    Very Low-Calorie Diets (VLCDs), 71–75, 110
Dietsmart.com, 232, 233
Dietz, William, 217
Doctors, 52–57
Downey, Morgan, 207, 208

Drug treatment
    as adjunct to therapy, 111, 122–126
    appetite suppressants, 112
    benefits of, 119–122
    candidates for, 115–117
    failures, 110
    fat blockers, 113
    "fixing" obesity with, 109–111
    limitations and risks of, 117–119
    medical advances in, 221–226
    nonprescription drugs, 176–183
    prescription drugs, 113–115
    stimulants, 112–113
    summary on, 126–127
Drugs and weight gain, 10, 16, 114

E

Eating disorders
    anorexia nervosa, 188, 191–192, 196
    binge eating disorder, 188–189, 194–195, 196
    bulimia nervosa, 188, 193–194
    night eating syndrome, 195–196
    treatment for, 196
Economics of obesity, 17–19
Ediets.com, 232, 233
Ehrlich, Paul, 209
Endocrinologists, 55
Endometrial cancer, 18, 24
Ephedra, 112–113, 178, 179, 180
Ephedrine, 112, 177–180
Estrogen, 23, 25
Exercise
    aerobic and anaerobic, 103
    children and, 215, 218
    consistent, 100–102
    diabetes and, 20–21
    importance of, 93, 94–97
    logs, 84, 97–98
    medical exam and, 97
    motivation and, 103–105
    self-assessment, 97–98
    target heart rate and, 99–100
    warm up and cool down, 103

F

Exercise physiologists, 60, 61–62, 66
Extreme obesity, 42, 45, 47

Fad dieting, 88–89
Families and sabotage, 198–199
Family physicians, 53
Fat
  defined, 27–28
  as living organ, 28
  uses for fat cells, 29–30
Fat blockers
  defined, 113
  orlistat (Xenical), 113, 115, 117, 118, 119, 120, 123, 126, 180, 181
Fat distribution, 36, 37
Fat magnets, 180–182
Fatty liver, 16, 23
Fenfluramine (Pondimin), 118, 122, 123, 163
Fen-phen, 110, 122–123, 126, 219
Fletcher, Anne, 92, 93, 94
Fluoxetine (Prozac), 114
Food log, 81–82, 106, 196
Food supplements
  fat magnets, 180–182
  FDA regulation of, 176–177
  medical advances in, 227–229
  questionable "diet aids," 177–180, 182–183
Foods, measuring, 82–83
Future treatments. *See* Medical advances

G

Gallbladder disease, 22, 24
Garvey, Steve, 181
Gastric bypass surgery
  benefits of, 144–145, 146
  complications, 143
  defined, 136–137
  diabetes and, 145, 146
  food restrictions after, 150–151
  paying for, 151, 208, 209
  Roux-en-Y, 137–139, 147
  rules to follow after, 148–149
  side effects, 144
  treatment after, 145–150
Gastric stimulator, 226
Gastroenterologists, 55
Genetic diseases, 10, 12–15
Genetics, 8, 9, 11, 187
Givens, Joanna, 30–33
Glazer, Gary, 119
Globesity, 17
Gordon, Dr. Judith, 107
Gout, 23

H

Heart disease
  bariatric surgery and, 146
  Dexatrim and, 178
  exercise and, 97
  fen-phen and, 110, 122–123
  obesity and, 18, 20–21
  sibutramine and, 118
  smoking and, 51
  in women, 36
Heart rate, target, 99–100
Hepatic steatosis, 23
Herbal medicines
  aristolochic acid in, 182–183
  FDA approval and, 176–177
  ma huang, 112–113, 179
  sales of, 176
High blood pressure. *See* Hypertension
Hill, Dr. James, 232, 234
Hsu, Dr. L.K. George, 196
Hunger awareness, 105–106
Hyperlipidemia, 21
Hypertension (high blood pressure)
  bariatric surgery and, 146
  obesity and, 18, 21–22
  sibutramine and, 118
  as sign of obesity, 37
Hypnotherapy, 167–171
Hypothalamus disorders, 10, 14–15
Hypothyroidism, 10, 13

I

Ideal body weight (IBW), 38–40, 73
Imaging tests, 49–50
Infertility, 23
Internet-based weight programs, 7, 230–233
Internists, 54

J

Jackson, Dr. Robert, 156
Jacobson, Michael, 238, 239
Jeffery, Robert, 235
Jenny Craig, 164, 165, 207

K

Kayman, Susan, 95, 105
Kelly, Walt, 35
Kral, Dr. John, 145, 149

L

Laparoscopically adjustable gastric band, 139, 151–154
Leibowitz, Sarah, 87
Leptin, 14, 15, 29, 221–223, 225
Leshner, Dr. Alan, 52
Lifestyle, 10, 11–12, 33
Liposuction, 154–156, 209
Liver disease, 23
Logs
 exercise, 84, 97–98
 food, 81–82, 106, 196
Low Calorie Diets (LCDs), 75–79

M

Ma huang, 112–113, 179
Magnuson, Dr. Thomas, 136, 142, 148, 151
Mallory, Georgeann, 133
Marlatt, Dr. G. Alan, 107
Marshall, Barry, 230
Mason, Dr. Edward, 136–137, 138
Mazindol (Mazanor, Sanorex), 113

Medical advances
 behavioral research, 232–236
 drug treatment, 221–226
 food supplements, 227–229
 Internet-based weight programs, 230–233
 medical devices, 226–227
 overview of, 219–220
 research on viruses, 229–230
Medical evaluation, 51–57
Medicare, 65–66, 208, 220
Medications and weight gain, 10, 16
Meridia (sibutramine), 115, 118, 120, 122, 123, 124, 126
Metformin, 13, 20–21
Mills, Don, 154
Morbid obesity, 42, 45
Muscle mass, 27, 40, 84

N

Native Americans, 9–10
Nestle, Marion, 238, 239
Nicotine, 15, 112. *See also* Smoking cessation
Niemtzow, Dr. Richard C., 172, 173, 175
Night eating syndrome, 195–196
Nutritionists, 60, 66

O

Obesity
 causes of, 8–16
 as complex condition, 2–8
 conditions associated with, 16–27
 as disease, 1–2
Olestra, 6, 220, 227, 228, 229
O'Neil, Patrick, 190
Orlistat (Xenical)
 chitosan versus, 180–181
 description of, 113, 115
 effectiveness of, 120, 123
 as fat blocker, 113
 FDA approval of, 115, 126
 side effects of, 117–118, 119

Osteoarthritis, 18, 22
Overweight versus obesity, 40, 42, 47

P

Pacific Islanders, 10
Pancreatic cancer, 26
Perkins, Kenneth, 53
Pets, overweight, 6–7
Phentermine, 115, 118, 119, 122, 123
Physicians, 52–57
Pima Indians, 9–10
Pinch test, 48–49
Plastic surgery, 154–156
Plateauing, 80–84
Pollack, Harold, 211
Polycystic ovary syndrome, 10, 13
Pool, Robert, 9, 10
Pories, Dr. W.J., 145, 150
Prader-Willi syndrome, 10, 12
Pregnancy
    appetite suppressants and, 118
    bariatric surgery and, 135
    breast-feeding, 39, 241
    Dexatrim and, 178
    diabetes and, 215
    infertility, miscarriage, and obesity, 23
    Very Low Calorie Diets and, 75
    weight gain during, 39
Prozac (fluoxetine), 114
Psychological issues
    behavioral issues, 105–108
    child abuse, 189, 197–198
    eating disorders, 191–196
    families and sabotage, 198–199
    Melissa's story, 199–206
    of obese people, 189–191
    stress, 188, 196–197
Pyruvate, 181–182, 183

R

RAND Institute, 27
Redux (dexfenfluramine), 118, 122, 123, 163

Richards, Dean, 174
Risk factors, 50–51
Rolls, Dr. Barbara, 229
Roux-en-Y gastric bypass, 137–139, 147

S

Satcher, Dr. David, 211, 236, 240
Scales, bathroom, 81
Scales, food, 82
Scopinaro, Dr. Nicola, 139
Set point theory, 84–87
Sherwood, Nancy, 235
Sibutramine (Meridia), 115, 118, 120, 122, 123, 124, 126
Skinfold caliper, 48–49
Sleep apnea, 23, 62, 63, 146
Slick, Grace, 109
Smith, Wayne, 156–159
Smoking cessation
    acupuncture and, 172
    bupropion (Wellbutrin) for, 114
    as cause of obesity, 10, 15, 51, 52–53, 112
    societal changes and, 241–242
Societal changes, 236–242
Society's treatment of the obese
    stereotypes, 206–207
    taxes, 207–209
Socioeconomic status, 51
Spiegel, Dr. Allen, 21
Steroids, 16, 30
Stimulants, 112–113
Strauss, Dr. Richard, 211
Stress, 96, 188, 196–197
Stroke, 22, 118, 178
Success
    defining, 79–80
    long-term, 91–94
    planning for, 87–90
Surgery
    benefits of, 144–145, 146
    candidates for, 133–136
    as choice of last resort, 129–130

food after, 150–151
laparoscopically adjustable gastric band, 139, 151–154, 156–159
liposuction, 154–156, 209
options for, 136–139
overview, 130–132
paying for, 151
recommended standards, 140–141
risks and side effects of, 139, 142–144
rules to follow after, 148–149
summary on, 159–160
treatment after, 145–150
Wayne Smith's story, 156–159
Susceptibility genes, 9, 11

T

Tax deductions, 207–209
Teas, dieter's, 177–178, 179, 182
Thompson, Tommy G., 20
Thromboembolism, 23–24
Thun, Dr. Michael, 24, 25, 26, 238
Total body water, 49
Treatment. *See* Complementary and alternative treatments; Diets; Drug treatment; Exercise; Medical advances; Surgery
Triglycerides, 28, 121
Tumor necrosis factor, 29
Type 2 diabetes
bariatric surgery and, 145, 146
childhood obesity and, 210, 215, 216
description of, 18, 19–20
Dexatrim and, 178
increase in, 19–20, 50
Joanna Givens' story, 30–33
Linda's story, 62–67, 188
liver disease and, 23
in Pima Indians, 10
as sign of obesity, 38, 97

V

Vertical banded gastroplasty (VBG), 137, 138, 144, 145
Very Low Calorie Diets (VLCDs), 71–75, 110
Virus research, 229–230

W

Waist circumference, 45–47
Walking, 101, 102, 104, 105
Weighing yourself, 81
Weight-management clinics, 57–62
Weight programs, Internet-based, 7, 230–233
Weight ranges, healthy, 40, 41
Weight Watchers, 88, 164, 201, 207, 233
Weil, Dr. Andrew, 163
Wellbutrin (bupropion), 114
Williamson, David, 225, 226
Williamson, Donald, 190
Wing, Dr. Rena, 234

X

Xenical (orlistat)
chitosan versus, 180–181
description of, 113, 115
effectiveness of, 120, 123
FDA approval of, 115, 126
side effects of, 117–118, 119

Y

Yanovski, Jack, 221, 223, 224
Yanovski, Susan, 195, 221, 223, 224

About the Authors

Lawrence J. Cheskin, M.D., is an associate professor at the Johns Hopkins Bloomberg School of Public Health and the Johns Hopkins School of Medicine. A gastroenterologist by training, he founded and directs the Johns Hopkins Weight Management Center, through which he has helped hundreds of individuals control their weight. He is the author of two other books, *Losing Weight for Good* and *3 Steps to Weight Loss*, as well as numerous studies in medical journals in the area of obesity and other nutritional concerns. He lives in Ellicott City, Maryland.

Ron Sauder is an editor and writer specializing in consumer health information. He is currently director of media relations for the health sciences at Emory University in Atlanta, Georgia. Prior to that he was managing editor for the Caregiver's Medical Guide, an online medical reference for family caregivers published by CareThere, Inc. As the first director of consumer health information for the Johns Hopkins University and Health System from 1996 to 1999, he helped to manage Johns Hopkins' participation in the pioneering consumer health information Web site, InteliHealth, a joint venture with Aetna U.S. Healthcare. He lives in Atlanta, Georgia.